Käthe

MW01292690

EARTH RADIATION

The Startling Discoveries of Harmful Effects on Health

**Results of Research
on more than 11,000 people in
over 3,000 apartments, houses,
and work places in 14 countries**

The recognition and correction of geopathic disturbances of sleep, health, and school performance

Foreword by Dr. Keith Mumby, MB, ChB.
Further Thoughts by John Living, Professional Engineer

Second Edition

Published by The Holistic Intuition Society
c/o Executive Secretary, John Living, Professional .Engineer
RR# 1 Site 9 Comp 6, Galiano Island, British Columbia, V0N 1P0 Canada
Telephone (250)539-5807 Toll Free Canada & USA: 1-866-369-7464

Check www.in2it.ca for any change in address

Käthe Bachler

EARTH

RADIATION

Second Edition

Published by The Holistic Intuition Society

For other books by John Living see:

www.in2it.ca/Books.htm

ISBN 978-0-9686323-5-2

Contents

Part II FAILURES IN SCHOOL POSSIBLY CAUSED BY GEOPATHIC ZONES OF DISTURBANCE AT HOME AND IN SCHOOL

Part III CASE HISTORIES AND STATISTICAL INFORMATION

Index to Case Histories

Motto for this Book

"Love alone will be the guide
whether we keep silent, whether we talk
whether we observe, whether we act..."
Gertrud Steinitz Metzler

The poet tells in her book 'The Rainbow-Bridge' what will help us in different situations to reach responsible, mature and appropriate decisions.

In the example of the Good Samaritan (Luke 10:25-37), all people are called upon to assist their fellow men in times of need, and especially in times of illness.

To convey the importance of the zones of disturbance is also a fulfillment of this command.

Note regarding the spelling used in this book

The original language of this book was German, which was translated by a lady in the USA - presumably into the USA brand of English. The first edition was then edited and published in England using the UK spellings.

John Living was educated in England, and now lives in Canada, which uses a mix-mash of UK-USA spellings.

English is always recognized as a 'Living Language'.

In so exercising his ownership rights and obligations, John Living uses his own variations in spelling, but has kept most medical words (not understood by him) as spelt in the first edition.

Translator's Foreword

The original German version of this book was brought to my attention by G. Duque-Mejia M.D. of Popayan, Colombia, South America, who was treating my 17 year old daughter for a severe illness, aggravated by years of her sleeping above a geopathic zone.

He himself had found the book valuable in his practice and had translated it from German into Spanish.

The German original contains an extensive bibliography which has not been translated for this English version, because the great majority of works cited have not themselves been translated into English. Interested German speaking readers may wish to refer to the German edition for this bibliography.

I chose to prepare an English translation because it represents to me an important area of research that is at present little known to physicians and laypersons in the United States.

It is my hope that physicians will consider geopathic conditions, as outlined in this book, when diagnosing and treating chronic or recurrent illnesses.

Teachers and parents might also keep in mind the possible role of geopathic zones when confronted with certain behavioral difficulties in children and adolescents.

We laymen, too, can benefit from increased cognizance of subtle influences on our functioning and well being, emotional as well as physical. This book, and the recommendations contained in it, provide helpful, simple tools for all of us.

Marianne Z. Gerhart

July, 1984

Preface

The author, Käthe Bachler, has been for many years a teacher and an educational leader in her field. She also has been active and innovative in the areas of various social problems.

She has always been eager and willing to extend herself to all the children in her care, but also to those with whom she did not have immediate contact.

She has always looked for ways to alleviate suffering and pain, and to do away with obstructions to well being.

And thus, it does not come as a surprise that she, a sensitive human being and also a woman trained in mathematics and science, was able to discover valuable methods in the use of the pendulum and the dowsing rod.

These particular methods have not enjoyed much attention from the scientific community until recently as a way to assist people in their pursuit of health and well being.

She has worked with energy and enthusiasm to explore the potential benefits of her work and to apply them usefully to everyday life.

Her main interest - and how could it be otherwise for a dedicated teacher - centred around the question of whether the failing academic performance of certain students might be caused by geopathic zones of disturbance.

Of course, she encountered ridicule and scorn, as have many innovative thinkers. Yet she also gained the support and interest of many teachers, physicians and psychologists, and the gratitude of the parents and the children to whom her findings meant help and relief.

When she was given a research grant from the School of Education in Salzburg, Austria, she was able to devote herself full time to this work. She wanted to find out whether there was a measurable connection between geopathy and academic failures in children of school age.

Heretofore, this had been a field regarded as charlatanism.

We now possess the results of her work. This book is recommended for skeptics as well as supporters. Maybe they, too, will become convinced that there are indeed geopathic influences, and that by eliminating them, some people can be helped immeasurably.

This work is particularly valuable because the author describes a great many cases she herself had observed and she illustrates them for us by drawing sketches and diagrams.

The credibility of her findings is therefore much enhanced.

Mathias Laireiter, Ph.D.

Superintendent of Schools, District of Salzburg, Austria

Foreword

It gives me great pleasure to introduce this book to the English speaking world.

It has been a best-seller for many years now in Germany and it deserves a far wider readership.

It will truly save lives and make many people happier and healthier than they would otherwise be.

Every idea has its time and I believe that the awareness of geopathic stress, as it is called, is timely and welcome to physicians and lay healers alike.

As a clinical ecologist and allergist I am greatly interested in the way in which our environment may cause illness and here is one of the most exciting, not to say sensational, discoveries yet.

It has been Miss Bachler's role to explore and verify the validity of this important phenomenon and communicate it skillfully and convincingly.

The book is the distillation of many years work, dowsing over 11,000 cases in over 3,000 homes in 14 countries, all catalogued, numbered and cross-referenced. The evidence she produces is overwhelming.

While it could not be called a scientific study as such, many of the techniques she uses fulfill all sensible criteria for excluding bias and preconditioning.

It has been my pleasure to attend cases with her and she works scrupulously and meticulously; she always works 'blind', that is, seeks to avoid any foreknowledge of the case which would jeopardize the integrity of the results.

Indeed in the first case she ever taught me to dowse, we were able to correctly deduce the patient's medical condition from dowsed information only.

Prediction, of course, is the fundamental basis of any workable scientific hypothesis.

Personally, I find the dowsers' case impossible to ignore.

The results are beneficial far too often to be explained by mere coincidence. In any case, quite apart from therapeutic effects, we now have a rapidly growing body of data in which scientific electronic instruments have been able to corroborate the dowsers findings.

In other words, there have been studies in which the 'bad places' indicated by a good dowser have been verified by readings on a geo-magnetometer.

It is a pity, in view of this precision, that dowsing does not enjoy a higher reputation in the English speaking countries.

Nevertheless, it may surprise the reader to know that it is used quite often at official levels here in the UK - but this isn't widely broadcast because of a certain inexplicable coyness about the matter.

One of my patients, a skilled dowser, has undertaken a number of commissions for the Ministry of Agriculture and Fisheries (such as finding swine fever corpses hidden by a farmer) and even the Ministry of Defense (finding horse carcasses infected with anthrax during research in World War Two), all with considerable success, I might add. Even the police, on occasion, have had recourse to the help of a dowser.

There are countless individual dowsing anecdotes that all add up to a tremendous body of support for this ancient and venerable art.

It would be an unwise physician who scoffed or ignored its findings - and a very insensitive one who failed to explore its potential to help his or her patients towards even better health.

Although the medical profession is quite backward in this respect here in the UK, it is worth pointing out that many doctors in Germany, Austria and France use dowsers in their health care programmes. Indeed, many of them undertake it personally.

Several of the authoritative figures from the history of dowsing were in fact medical doctors.

Just such a person was Dr. Manfred Curry, who discovered the existence of the dangerous network of rays named after him, which is referred to frequently in this book - the Curry Net.

Possibly the most exciting aspect of geopathic stress is the possibility that it might be a significant factor in the causation of cancer. If so, we stand on the brink of a new era in medicine and I for one can hardly wait !

I offer a simple but challenging diagram for perusal. It is the plan of a small German town and on it are marked the dangerous rays detected by a skilled dowser physician.

Also marked are the beds of everyone in that town who had died of cancer. As you can see, all of them fall where the dowser predicted there was danger.

Remember, he carried out his study BEFORE identifying the cancer beds.

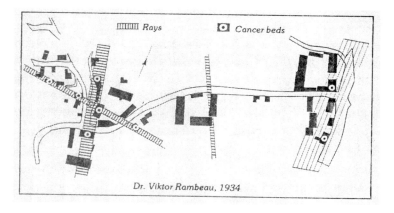

Dr. Viktor Rambeau, 1934

Convincing ? I think so.

The reader is also referred to the cases on pages 200-209 of this book.

But the contribution of Käthe Bachler has been to show that the effect is much wider than just cancer. Chronic illness of all kinds may respond to sleeping in a safer place.

Here is her testimony, a great gift to Mankind. It was hard-won knowledge: searching for harmful radiation often has a damaging effect on the dowser, and she became extremely ill at times and might easily have died, but for the support of those around her.

Nevertheless, she survived to deliver her message to the world and indeed is again formidably healthy and energetic, despite her advancing years.

It is my privilege to have been befriended by her, and I am thankful for this small role in making her work more widely known.

Dr Keith Mumby

Manchester, England, 1988

2007: Update on Dr Mumby: www.scott-mumby.com

Dr Keith Scott-Mumby MB ChB, MD, PhD, FRCP (Medicina Alternativa) is currently living in Palm Springs, California

Professional status:

Member of the Royal Society of Medicine UK (elected-only membership)

Founder member, the British Society for Nutrition, Allergy and Environmental Medicine

Medical Advisor, board of 'What Doctors Don't Tell You' (journal)

Scientific and medical advisor to the British Society for Homotoxicology

Member American Academy of Anti-Ageing Medicine (A4M)

Certified member of American College for the Advancement of Medicine

Professor of Nutrition (visiting) Open International University for Complementary Medicines, Colombo, Sri Lanka

Professor of Bio-Energy Medicine, Capital University for Integrative Medicine, Washington DC.

Dr Scott-Mumby's Career:

"My early years were controversial. That always happens with new advances in thinking and science. In the early 1980s, I was called a quack by certain hardcore orthodox doctors in my home town. Food allergy was called 'Mumby-Jumbo' at the local city hospital.

Yet by the end of the 80s, physicians were beginning to sneak either themselves or their wives into my clinic as patients. By the end of the 90s even the senior specialists were turning up as patients too. Eventually the tide turned and my former critics were being interviewed and admitting that what I had said over a decade before was true."

"It was gratifying that in 1994 the UK Government Health Officer released an official communiqué, stating that chemicals in traffic fumes could sensitize individuals to allergens; I had been saying it for years and been scoffed at."

"By the end of the 1990s, matters had moved on to the point where the National Health Service (the UK government social medicine system) were buying my anti-allergy prescription formulas for patients. To have gone from quack to 'official' in less than 20 years is fast progress in medical science !"

"As a recognized expert in alternative health matters, my name became attached to many medical breakthroughs."

"By 1990 the media were calling me the 'Number One Allergy Detective', the name which finally stuck. This in acknowledgement of the many extraordinary allergies I discovered on individuals. This resulted in frequent radio and TV appearances, to discuss such matters, which intrigued the public greatly."

"In 2005 I was elected as a Fellow of the Royal College of Practitioners and became associate professor at the Capital University for Integrative Medicine in Washington DC."

Professional Publications

The Food Allergy Plan (Unwins 1985)
Allergies: What Everyone Should Know (Unwins 1986)
The Allergy Handbook (Thorsons 1988)
The Poisoned Tree (Sidgwick & Jackson, and Pan Paperback 1990)
The Complete Guide to Food Allergy and Environmental Illness
(Thorsons 1993)
Virtual Medicine (Thorsons 1999), Timpanogos Publishing (2004)
Diet Wise: Let your body choose the food, Timpanogos (2007)
(see www.dietwisebook.com)

Troubled by Dowsing ?

A note from the Archbishop of Salzburg.

"Clemency supposes good nature !" This theological saying is as valid today as it always was. In our time, people are subject to many more detrimental environmental forces than in former times.

All right-minded men and women are called upon to try to help each other overcome these adverse influences.

Anyone who is able should strive to help people preserve a sound body and soul or to win it back again.

Ms. Käthe Bachler, a believer and practicing Christian, endeavours to live a good everyday life. With her dowsing instruments she can find the 'good places' and has thus helped many people, as well as several priests and sisters of our archdiocese.

All good things can however be abused and thus also the work with rod and pendulum. Therefore the Church warns people not to use these instruments for occult experiments.

We draw attention to the fact that work with a rod and pendulum can be dangerous if arrogance, curiosity, evil thoughts or greed are the sole motive.

If however a Christian wants to do God's will and protects himself with prayers when doing radiaesthesic works and uses his or her instruments only in a helping way, based on love, when examining houses and finding water, then this work is blessed by the Church (Decree of 26 March 1942).

In this sense I can recommend unreservedly and warmly to believing Christians the work of Ms. Käthe Bachler and especially her book 'The Startling Discoveries of a Dowser', now translated into English as 'Earth Radiation'.

Dr. Karl Berg
Archbishop of Salzburg

Acknowledgements

With all my heart, I would like to thank Marianne Gerhart for preparing this English translation of my book. Also my many friends in England who have paved the way for my work, particularly Ilse Pope.

Above all, I want to thank Dr. Keith Mumby, an exceptional physician, for overseeing the publication of this work. He is the first doctor in England to grasp the full importance of my discoveries and I have no doubt that it is his vision, as well as mine, to see that knowledge of the potential harmful effects of earth radiation is spread throughout the world.

With the publisher's permission, I would like to make a comment on the association between science and religion.

At the beginning of my researches I held the misguided belief that it was important to keep these two separate.

Now I see things differently.

In my view, only when the scientific dowser feels a responsibility towards God and is humble and full of love towards his fellow man, will dowsing succeed.

Without guidance from above, the dowser will fall into error and may thus do harm to himself and others.

Properly carried out, dowsing is a Divine service to one's fellows.

This, I believe, is the answer to the criticism, sometimes voiced, that dowsing is a dark and sinister force.

A good dowser is following God' s will.

This is important for all dowsers to understand, no matter what his or her religion.

Done in such a spirit, the dowser's work will be of benefit to all.

This is my wish for the great family of Man !

Käthe Bachler
Manchester, England, 1988.

Introduction

This book serves as a general and important source of information for everyone. It deals with two major detrimental effects of our environment.

In the countryside near Salzburg, little Manfred suffered from severe asthma. His father told me, *"The doctor gave strong medication, but it really did not help. Finally, he told us that the child was allergic to something in his environment. Since I had heard of the theory about the negative influences of the earth on health, I simply pushed my child's bed back into another corner of the room. He never had another attack".*

A month later I had occasion to examine this house thoroughly (Case# 1177, page 130). I ascertained that the first place where Manfred slept stood above an underground water current, as well as a Curry crossing, and that the subsequent place was indeed free of these negative influences. In other words, it was a neutral place.

Yes, indeed; Manfred suffered from 'allergies to the earth' and he could get well only after he was no longer exposed to these damaging influences.

What do I mean by 'allergies to the earth' ?

It is a particularly high sensitivity in regard to influences which originate in the deeper parts of the earth itself. Life is manifold. We are exposed to many different influences, good and bad.

Many factors can disturb health and well being, like weather changes, one's lifestyle, a bad diet and infections. Many of these factors can be eliminated, once recognized.

In addition, there are other environmental factors less familiar to most people, such as the influences from the earth itself - that is geopathic influences.

I want to report about these geopathic influences, since very few facts and conclusions have been presented in this area.

It would be of great value for people to know more about them, especially since much energy could be preserved, much suffering alleviated, much emotional turmoil eased, and many people could lead a useful and happy life, if those damaging influences could be removed from their lives.

I have always been a person who likes to use her critical faculties, and who likes to get to the bottom of things.

Thus, when I came into contact with dowsing, I made the decision to research this phenomenon. As a mathematician I was eager to make a situation more real by doing a sketch or a drawing.

Physicians became interested in my work, I have given many public lectures about geopathic influences, and people have urged me to put my experiences and conclusions into book form.

Thus, this factual report has its origin in the spoken word, and the style of the book is therefore somewhat informal and personal.

I urge you to read the book critically, even with a skeptical mind, but without prejudice or intolerance. Please approach this book with the openness so necessary for this kind of subject which heretofore has not been explored.

After you have finished the book, you will have to concede that the thousands of case histories could not possibly be based on mere coincidences, but that there must be deeper connections present which have not yet been researched or understood.

Also, please do not take words out of context. Refrain from judging the book until you have read it though.

Reading it partially may cause misunderstandings. Some of the repetitions have to do with the way the book was put together and I ask for your indulgence. All of my statements can be backed by evidence.

I want to thank God first and foremost for having given me the gift of sensitivity, without which I could never have succeeded as a dowser.

And then I want to thank the courageous pioneers of the art of dowsing all over the world, and in particular those in Salzburg, Austria, who invited me in 1969 to an excursion into the Salzburg Moors.

There I experienced my first reaction of the dowsing rod.

After a year of intensive work I met the successful Austrian dowser Adolf Flachenegger. This master and outstanding teacher examined me, approved my work and took me into the inner circle of the Austrian dowsers. I owe him and the group of friends concerned with the progress of dowsing a wealth of gratitude.

I also want to express my appreciation and gratitude to Dr. R. von Kolitcher for so many valuable suggestions and for encouragement to engage in scientific research.

He urged me to use my proven abilities to help people, and to use my talent in finding geopathic zones to support physicians in their medical practice.

And I thank all those physicians who had confidence in me, and who used my assistance in their most difficult cases by having me point out the damaging environmental influences.

I thank the school district for its open-mindedness, especially Dr. Mathias Laireiter, and I thank the Pedagogical Institute in Salzburg for the assignment 'Research into the connections between geopathic zones of disturbances and the academic failures in school children'.

I am also thankful for all the people who took the trouble to tell me about the improvement in their condition, especially those who wrote to me about it.

And also to the schoolchildren who were so happy to tell me right after their beds had been moved, how much better they felt and how much better they could sleep at night.

It is my sincere desire that the realizations on which this book is based will be instrumental in giving help and hope to the many people who have suffered from illness and depressions.

I am thinking especially of children who are unable to bring about a change without the help and understanding of the adults around them.

Käthe Bachler

Hallein, Salzburg, Austria, 1976

Abbreviations and Symbols

Sleeping area as found

Sleeping area as recommended or, as sometimes was the case, as it was found already to be 'good'.

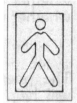

Male

Female

C: Curry lines (zone of disturbance named after Manfred Curry, M.D.)

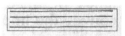

W: Water currents

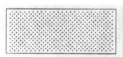

CxC: Curry Crossing

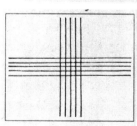

WxW: Water Crossing

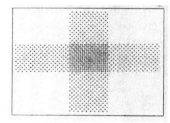

Part I - GENERAL INTRODUCTION

1. Rays, Emanations from the Earth;
Sensitivity to Emanations from the Earth.

The existence of rays and radiation is an indisputable fact. We think of visible light rays from the sun, heat rays, Roentgen rays or X rays, the radioactive decay radiations from radium, infrared and ultraviolet rays, radio and television rays, rays of radar, and cosmic rays.

There also exist 'Earth Rays' (including emanations from the earth above subterranean running water).

It is not understood exactly how they come into existence.

Some experts believe that they are secondary radiations caused by cosmic rays striking the subterranean water; others maintain that they are diffuse emanations from the inside of the earth, which become concentrated and directed upward by subterranean water currents.

It is also an indisputable fact that many of the rays mentioned above exert a damaging influence on humans; no reasonably informed person will argue that point.

The 'emanations from the earth', too, have a damaging effect.

I dare make this pronouncement because of my vast experience in this particular area of research. In the latter part of the book, dealing with case histories and practical explanations, I will attempt to prove this point.

It is known that some people have a 'sixth sense' for rays, even though they are invisible.

This ability to perceive rays we call 'sensitivity'.

It is unfortunate that the majority of people have lost this sensitivity.

Our twentieth-century lifestyle is partially to blame, but also the fact that many people do not trust their 'sensitivity' and even feel that it needs to be suppressed and denied.

Yet, in recent years we have recognized that 'sensitivity' in regard to various natural phenomena can be a most helpful and valuable protection.

It seems as though people have actually become more sensitive in recent times.

There are people - small children in particular - who possess this sensitivity to a high degree.

They are able to ascertain with great accuracy the different kinds of radiation with the aid of a pendulum or dowsing rod.

In both sexes we find people whose sensitivity is highly developed, and they tend to have an innate talent in regard to the use of the pendulum or dowsing rod.

The area concerned with earth rays and the sensitivity to it is called 'Dowsing' in English, or 'Radiesthesia' in many other languages.

These particular people are sensitive physically as well as emotionally.

They show a tendency to be 'thin-skinned', serious-minded, tactful, altruistic, willing to put themselves out for others, but also easily hurt and offended.

Members of the helping professions frequently show a high degree of this kind of sensitivity.

Many people showed me their favourite place in the living room or maybe in the kitchen.

And they could also indicate which bed they particularly liked to sleep in.

Invariably, I found these to be 'good' places.

These people had preserved their original sensitivity.

There already exists photographic proof for the phenomenon of radiesthesia.

It was first advanced by the physicist Dr. Paul Dobler from Stuttgart, Germany.

A teacher of physics, Helmuth Boehm, substantiated these facts later at the 1973 Austrian Congress for Radiesthesia with a paper entitled 'Infrared Photography in the Service of Radiesthesia'.

2. How do Plants & Animals React to Subterranean Water ?

There are two known groups of organisms: those who avoid the different rays, and those who seek them out.

'Ray Avoiders' are those organisms which cannot tolerate the energy emanating from the subterranean waters and thus avoid them or flee from them.

If that is impossible, they become weak or sick.

Plants growing in the wild will usually only germinate in those areas which possess favourable conditions.

Cultivated plants have a tendency to avoid areas not to their liking by growing crookedly (often against the direction of the wind), and if that does not work, they become sick (like a cancerous tree above a water current), or they die (like a lilac above a water crossing, or some bushes in a red currant hedge).

Apple and pear trees have the most aversion to these terrestrial rays, as do nut trees, currant bushes, lilacs and sunflowers.

In the forest it is the beech trees and the linden trees (both said to be good protection in case of electrical storms) that avoid terrestrial radiation, and among indoor plants, it is the begonias, the azaleas, and the different cacti.

'Ray Seekers' are those plants and animals that actually thrive above subterranean water and enjoy being there.

Cherry trees, plum, nectarine, peach, elderberry trees, and mistletoes are all 'ray seekers'. (From a paper by Professor I. Cracmar: 'A remedy made from mistletoe is used in case of radiation illness'.)

In the forest it is known that oak trees and fir trees have an affinity for terrestrial rays (both trees should be avoided in case of lightning), as do asparagus and aralia.

Case# 1587a: A Look at an Orchard

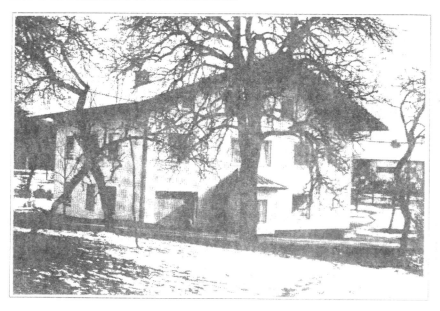

a   b   c

a.   Apple tree, 50 years old, was planted above a water current and therefore has grown bent and crooked.

      Only the tip which hangs over a 'radiation free' spot bears a few apples.

b.   The pear tree stands on a radiation-free place.

      It grew tall, strong and straight and bears much fruit.

c.   The apple tree above the crossing of two water currents is 'cancerous' and has big lumps and bulges on its trunk.

      This stunted tree has never borne any fruit.

Whenever a tree does poorly or dies, one might consider planting in its place a type of tree which is known to thrive under the opposite conditions.

We also know that potatoes and other vegetables will rot when stored in cellars exposed to harmful subterranean rays.

Jams and jellies will start going mouldy, and wine will not mature.

In March 1977, I was asked by Dr. Anton Schneider, Professor at the Trade School in Rosenheim, Bavaria, to participate as a dowser in a workshop on geobiology and its role in regard to building codes and healthful living spaces.

My special task was to examine a plot in a forest nearby in order to study diseases of trees in connection with 'terrestrial rays'.

As it turned out, the trees which were most severely damaged stood exactly above those areas which registered the greatest terrestrial radiation.

Those trees suffered from total loss of their bark, were infested by bark beetles, and showed cancerous growth.

Animals in the wild seek out the places which are comfortable for their species. Domesticated animals are not so fortunate. The 'ray avoiders' try to get away from the water currents by standing lopsided, and if that is not possible, they become ill.

The animals who will flee from rays are dogs, horses, cows, pigs (there is a German saying 'no pig can tolerate this'), chickens and birds. Even an otherwise obedient dog will not heed his master's command if ordered to lie on a radiated spot.

Case# 122

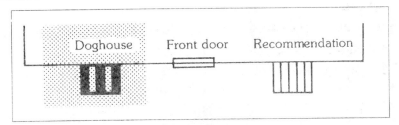

One day I observed a doghouse above a water current.

When I mentioned that I thought the dog would not be happy there the woman replied: *"He never goes in there anyway. He prefers the cement floor by the front door".*

The doghouse was immediately moved to an area free of disturbing rays, and the dog has slept there ever since and seems to be content.

Infertility and abortion of domesticated animals is caused in many instances by a radiated location which they cannot escape, as in cases of horses, cattle and pigs.

There was one particular spot in a cowshed, a farmer's wife observed, where every single cow became ill and many of them died. Thus, she asked me for an investigation.

The farmer himself said:

"I don't believe that water so deep in the ground can harm a big cow. I won't tell you where the sick cow usually lies" (at that time all fifteen cows were lying down at their stalls) *"and I am curious whether you can find it with your dowsing rod".*

But when my dowsing rod turned sharply at the second turn he exclaimed, *"You are correct, that's where the sick cow is lying. I would not have believed it."*

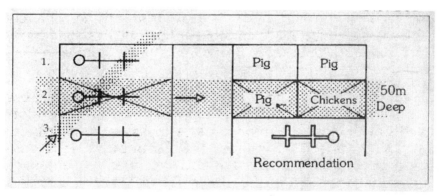

He further reported:

"Over there, where you believe the water current to continue, we lost a pig and also three chickens this year, without any reason at all. In the other two pigsties the animals always do very well".

<u>Case# 181</u>

There are two German sayings, 'Swallows bring good luck to a house', and 'The stork brings the babies'. Those are old sayings based on centuries of observation.

<u>Birds will only nest where there is no radiation from the earth</u>. And those are the places where people, too, will feel well, and where women will bear healthy children.

Be sure to hang your birdhouses on trees which will only grow on radiation free spots, such as on a healthy apple or pear tree !

'Rayseekers' are cats, bees, ants, insects, bacteria and parasites.

Cats will prefer the crossing of two water currents, or at least a strongly radiated area.

Ants and wild bees will always be found above the crossing of two underground water currents.

A psychology student told me of an old Bavarian custom.

Before the groundbreaking took place for building a house, an anthill was put onto the ground - presumably in the exact spot where the bedroom was planned.

Only if the ants moved away, which would indicate a location free of radiation, would the building proceed as planned.

Otherwise, another spot would be tried.

Domesticated bees yield much more honey above a radiated area, and wild bees will always swarm above a water current crossing.

Bacteria and parasites will infect people already weakened from sleeping above a radiated area and they will multiply rapidly.

That is also true of the tubercle bacillus.

This chapter is based on the writings of Arnold Flachenegger, published thirty years ago, whose observations I have been able to substantiate in many cases.

Lightning will strike only where two water currents cross at a substantial difference in depth.

Dr. Deibel, an attorney from Munich, Germany, has established that connection, after having examined 100 farmhouses and buildings.

A friend told me that this fact was explained to him forty years ago at the University of Vienna, during a physics lecture.

I was able to make the same observation in fourteen cases.

Spontaneous combustion of haystacks, or the dust explosion of stored coal, usually takes place above such water crossings.

3. What Reaction do People Have to Subterranean Water ?

Babies and small children have an innate sensitivity to subterranean radiation, and they instinctively attempt to avoid those areas, even while asleep.

A young mother, the wife of a physicist, observed her ten month old son Severin sitting up in bed about two minutes after he fell asleep, acting as though he 'smelled' something, and then falling down at a spot which turned out to be free of harmful influences. There he slept peacefully, lying diagonally in his crib (1316 b).

I have observed repeatedly that infants and small children roll away from certain places in the bed or crib in their sleep. Sensitive school children, adolescents, and some adults will instinctively avoid those areas whenever possible, in bed as well as elsewhere. I want to cite just a few cases:

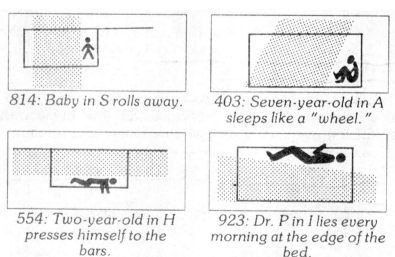

814: Baby in S rolls away.

403: Seven-year-old in A sleeps like a "wheel."

554: Two-year-old in H presses himself to the bars.

923: Dr. P in I lies every morning at the edge of the bed.

Some children's need to avoid the disturbing subterranean influences goes so far that they fall out of bed with all of their blankets. Many continue sleeping on the floor.

In more than a thousand cases I was able to point out the fact that infants and toddlers cry and toss restlessly only if they are lying on radiated places.

Fortunate is the infant who is then carried around when his mother takes pity on him. Unfortunate is the child who might even be tied to the bed 'so it will not fall out' or stand up all the time.

The first year of life is of utmost importance for our emotional development. If no help is forthcoming, despite desperate crying and screaming, the baby might later get sick, emotionally and physically. Those are often the people who become bitter and withdrawn in later life.

I have an urgent request to all of my readers: whenever you hear of a baby which cries all the time, suggest to the parents a change of place of the basket, cradle, or the crib, for better or worse. Or have a dog select the best place for the child (wherever the dog lies down is the very best spot). Or have them use the 'Location Test' (see page 212).

Many small children, but also sensitive children of school age, flee from their own radiated beds to those of their parents or siblings, usually without even waking up.

However, that solution presupposes that the parents or siblings have beds which are free of radiation, or are at least less disadvantaged.

I can substantiate these claims with evidence which I have gathered over the years.

Case# 1089: Bruno flees from his bed to his brother in his sleep.

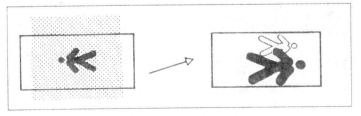

Many sensitive adults walk back and forth in their rooms at night for hours at a time, because they cannot stand it in their beds.

They have no idea why this is so. During full moon the effects of subterranean water are especially intense, and some people will sleepwalk at that time (Case# 632) because they are literally driven out of bed.

People unable to avoid these disturbance zones, and who are therefore exposed to their damaging influence all the time, will experience a marked decrease in their resistance to infection. The first symptoms tend to be some form of insomnia, tiredness and a 'run down' feeling in the morning, and eventually the emergence of real illness.

To avoid misunderstandings, I want to clarify the following: Subterranean water currents and other disturbance factors are not to be considered pathogenic agents as such, as are viruses or bacteria, but they tend to weaken the resistance to illness to a considerable degree.

The person who has lived above such disturbance zones over a long period of time will use so much energy to combat their influences that not much resistance is left to combat the illnesses which confront them at all times.

At the same time, we can strengthen our resistance which comes from the cosmos by living a healthful life and by eliminating damaging and harmful influences from our environment.

An attempt to illustrate my observations

1. Those people who sleep and work in areas entirely 'free of radiation' possess a marked resistance 'R'. Illness 'I' remains sub-acute because it cannot develop fully, even though other harmful influences might be present.

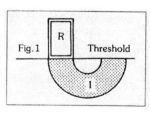

Fig. 1   R   Threshold   I

I have noticed many times, for example, that those children will not catch the flu, even though their siblings come down with it. However, only one person out of ten has the good fortune to be living in an environment totally free of radiation.

Those people enjoy good health and well-being often until a ripe old age.

2. Those people whose sleep and working spaces are only minimally influenced by disturbance zones will still feel well most of the time.

Yet their resistance is being drained, and illness will 'show up' at times - even more so, if additional disturbing influences are also present.

The resistance 'R' now moves below the threshold, while the illness 'I' moves above.   Note figure 2.

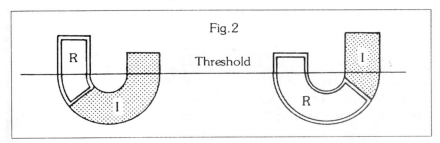

Fig.2

Threshold

3. People whose sleeping place and/or working space lies directly above a strongly radiated zone (for example, over several disturbance zones) often lose all of their resistance.

Then we see a 'taking over' of illness. And the more other negative influences are present the more the illness will take over.   See Figure 3.

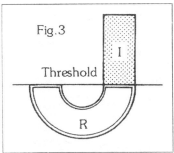

Fig.3

Threshold

Especially in our days of pollution everywhere, over which we can exert so little influence, we cannot afford to weaken our resistance even more by not heeding the negative influences which emanate from the earth.

4. Locating the Subterranean Water Currents

(a). Subterranean water currents can be located with scientific instruments: field intensity measuring instruments, low frequency sound probes, geiger counters, neutron counters, etc.

Some of these instruments are rather awkward to handle and are still very expensive.

(b). Results can be obtained much more simply, less expensively, and faster. We can get results with the dowsing rod as long as a sensitive person handles it.

The 'wooden fork' (that is, a bent branch), a staff (the 'staff of Moses'), a wire sling, and others are all forms of the dowsing rod.

In several instances, I had my own results with the dowsing rod confirmed by the objective methods that a modern apparatus affords.

As proof I submit an excerpt from a letter of a family from Bonn, Germany, dated January 10, 1981:

"A staff member of the Institute for Construction Biology in Rosenheim examined our bedroom and living room with an electrical device. Your conclusions were confirmed."

In the ancient Chinese culture it was required. that the location of a prospective house be examined with a dowsing rod before the house was built.

The Chinese emperor Yu wrote the first book about dowsing and the dowsing rod in 2000 B.C. In carved relief, he is pictured holding a dowsing rod.

To look for water with a dowsing rod is an old and well-known practice. Many of the spas were discovered that way. Professor Benedict from the University of Vienna explains dowsing as a phenomenon of physics.

According to him the bipolar (positive and negative) sides of the body are closed in an 'emanation stream' through the dowsing rod.

The characteristic 'turning of the rod' occurs at the moment jhe dowser walks over the field of disturbance.

Russia considers dowsing a legitimate field for scientific study. A scientific committee declared 'the dowsing rod is the simplest physical instrument of all electro-physical instruments imaginable'.

In the geological institutes in Moscow and Leningrad, radiesthesia is being studied by geologists, geophysicists and physiologists.

Rather than merely observe dowsers, the scientists (among them Nikolai Sotschewanow) use the pendulum and the dowsing rod themselves.

In other parts of the world we also find scientists who use the dowsing rod as a valuable tool in their work.

I did some collaborative work with the Austrian hydrogeologist Professor Emil Worsch, Ph.D., and our results agreed.

(c). A sensitive person can determine the course of an underground water current also with a pendulum. The pendulum, usually a pointed object that hangs from a little chain or thread, will make various motions - circles, ellipses, or straight lines.

The Catholic priest Abbe Mermet in Switzerland is considered a leader in the use of a pendulum. In his book 'The Pendulum: A Scientific Instrument', he takes issue with the notion that to 'pendel' constitutes quackery.

Abbe Mermet has found wells for many villages and has examined many apartments and buildings. Examining living quarters for subterranean water currents has validity and is neither magic or superstition.

(d). There are even some exceptional people who are able to detect running water in the earth by simply using their hands. They hold the palm of the hand toward the ground and as they approach subterranean water, they feel slight shivers, or a sensation of 'pins and needles', a pulling sensation, or even mild pain.

Damp spots on the wall, cracks in the walls or cement floors, as well as crumbling of walls and other parts of the house may also be signs of underground currents.

5. Other Influences from the Earth

(a). Physicists tell us that the globe is surrounded by its own field of rays, waves, and energy, the so called earth field or earth magnetic field. These are natural, harmonious, good rays, and we need them to sustain life.

However, at certain locations, plains, strips or zones, we find these fields of rays to be disturbed or dislocated.

There we find disharmonious, harmful rays. These interfering rays are often called 'earth rays'. The areas where these earth rays are found we will call 'zones of disturbance' or 'areas of irritation'.

Their causes can be subterranean or underground water courses, geological cracks or faults, hollow spaces, etc., or 'global grids', which have been re-discovered within the past few decades.

These have become more recognized because their effective intensities have increased since our environment - especially our houses - have become so invaded by electro-magnetic rays.

Eleven types of influences and disturbances can be identified with the aid of the pendulum or the dowsing rod.

This practice was common in the Middle Ages when prospecting for gold, silver, copper and iron. In recent years these instruments have been used to locate coal and iron.

The Austrian oilfield Zistersdorf was found with the use of the dowsing rod by Major Friedrich Musil. I myself can distinguish between the different global grids, and I am able to find them with the dowsing rod.

At a meeting for dowsers in November 1970, I volunteered for one experiment of this nature, and was successful on the first try.

(b). My extensive practical work with the dowsing rod has made me aware of the effect that daily exposure to a 'global grid' can have on a normally sensitive person.

This grid is known by the name of 'Curry net' in recognition of the work done by Manfred Curry, M.D.

Dr. Curry was the director of the Medical-Bioclimatic Institute in Riederau, and he conducted many experiments on the influence of weather and geological conditions on humans.

In his book 'The Key to Life' he distinguishes the W-type, the person who is sensitive to warmth (sympaticotonic - E. Hartmann, M.D.) and the person who is sensitive to cold (vagotonic - E. Hartmann, M.D.).

In the publication for practical medical science, 'Hippocrates', Dr. Curry published another scientific work, 'Identification of Responses Based on Climatic Influences, Through Measurements of Energies Emanating from the Body and Their Relation to Cancer' (reprinted by Herold Publications, Munich 71, 1981, under the name of 'Curry - Grid').

Dr.Curry advanced the theory that people send a pattern of waves, which differs uniquely from person to person.

The length of these waves he calls the 'reaction distance' or 'response interval'. Dr. Helmuth Boehm explained Dr. Curry's theories at a seminar for dowsers in 1974 as follows:

W-type ('sensitive to warmth' type, especially to warm alpine wind).

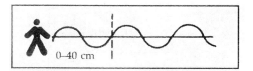

0–40 cm

MW (mixed types) MC

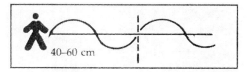

40–60 cm

C-type ('sensitive to cold' type, especially to cold weather fronts)

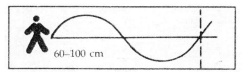

60–100 cm

The response interval is variable, which means it can change at any time. Different factors can cause it to shorten or lengthen.

Shortening of the response interval can be caused by:
- drugs causing dilation of blood vessels;
- warm weather;
- rays (like infrared rays);
- 'discharging' geological intersections;
- certain forms of nutrition.

Lengthening of the response interval can be caused by:
- vasoconstrictive drugs;
- cold weather;
- rays (for instance radioactive rays);
- 'charging' geological intersections;
- certain forms of nutrition.

Different types of people should strive toward the ideal response interval, which is in the middle range (50cm).

Zones of geopathic disturbance, according to Dr. Curry, influence the response interval even in the absence of any other factor. This is particularly true for the subterranean water crossings and other geological intersections.

Dr. Curry claims that cancer is usually present when the response interval becomes longer than 100cm.

In the same publication 'Hippocrates' Dr. Curry published another article: 'The Reaction System as Pathogenic Factors'. There he addresses himself primarily to the 'zones of disturbance grid'. I recommend these articles very highly. (They were published by Herold Publications, Munich 71 in 1981 under the title of the 'Curry - Grid'.)

I follow the course of this grid exactly whenever I examine any living quarters with the dowsing rod, and I have found it to be damaging to people's health.

These zones of disturbance are found to run along the intermediate compass points, that is, NE - SW and SE - NW.

11½ to 13.12 feet

In Central Europe, where Austria has a latitude of N.48, the grid lines can usually be found separated by a distance of 3.5 to 4 metres.

In the more northern countries, we find the grid lines closer together - in Northern Germany, for instance in Emden at the North Sea (53 degrees latitude), I found them at a distance of 2.75 to 3 metres.

In Bolivia, however, which is so much closer to the equator (17 degrees latitude), I found the separation of lines at 4.5 to 5 metres. I examined the hospital in El Chochis and there I was able to draw a fairly large area very accurately.

14¾′ to 16.4′

I feel each line or strip to be about 75cm. wide, but their width varies, according to the weather.

29½″

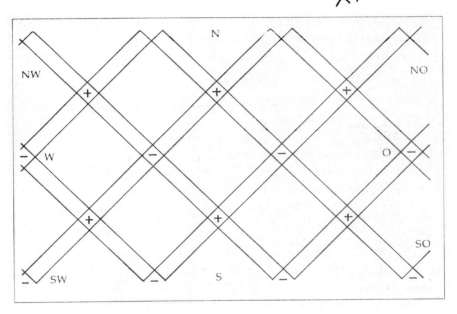

Dr. Curry used various instruments to measure the influences above the grid.

He distinguished two kinds of intersections of lines within the net.

One kind has a charging effect (+), which lengthens the response interval (individual human wavelength pattern) of a person.

The other kind has a discharging effect (-), which shortens the response interval. These are arranged in a regular, alternating array. He found that positive or charging intersections enhanced cell enlargement and cell proliferation, even to the point of cancerous growth.

On the other hand, negatively charged intersections enhanced inflammations. He recorded many of these findings and measurements in the form of graphs and tabulations. These intersections will be known as 'Curry crossings'.

Although the influences of the subterranean water currents have been known for a long time, it seems the global grid has only recently begun to be recognized as exercising harmful effects on people.

This fact may be connected with the general weakening of our health due to our modern lifestyle. Yet, not everyone is equally sensitive.

I have observed many people react to the presence of the Curry net with increased nervousness. The net seems to affect the vegetative nervous system.

By themselves, the lines or bands have little negative effect. Only above the Curry crossings or at positions where the net meets with subterranean water currents do we find that people suffer from trembling, spasms, at times even fainting.

I have observed and recorded several such cases, and all of them were related to these zones of disturbance. Some people have the sensation of electricity when above curry crossing.

One particularly sensitive eleven year old boy said, *"I feel as though lightning were hitting me"* (Case# 160).

Dr. Curry, and later on Dr. Petschke, did many measurements of blood sedimentation rates and found the results differed depending on whether the experiment was conducted on neutral ground or above a zone of disturbance.

A Note of Explanation:

I use the expression 'zone of disturbance' most of the time, but sometimes I will also use the term 'zone of interference', 'lines of interference', 'pathogenic zone', or 'radiated location or place'. With all these terms, I address myself to subterranean water currents as well as Curry lines, unless I mention one source or another specifically.

References to 'change of bed' always refer to the moving of the bed to a 'good place', namely, away from a zone of disturbance.

How can the dowser or the 'pendulist' (a person who uses the pendulum) distinguish between the different 'earth rays', that is, between the different kinds of radiating effects from the earth ?

I prefer to use the analogy of radio and television.

The desired reception comes about by carefully tuning the receiver to a desired frequency.

A sensitive person or a person who has inborn talent for the use of the pendulum or the dowsing rod and who in general is in tune with himself and the world around him can indeed tune into the different earth rays.

He will simply say to himself: *"I want to be sensitive to subterranean water currents, and I want to exclude any other form of geological interference".*

On another occasion he might want to single out the Curry net, or whatever else might be important to him at that time.

The ability to formulate one's intention precisely, without any mental effort, is the prerequisite to success.

The beginner, however, should not set his goals too high, and he should not become discouraged when difficulties ensue.

The serious student must seek the guidance of an experienced dowser or must attend workshops to gain practical experience under the proper instruction.

This is advisable also in view of the fact that the beginner needs to learn some precautionary measures so as not to jeopardize his own health.

Of course, not all dowsers have the time to draw up plans and make exact diagrams of all the currents and grids when they examine living quarters.

I needed to do this work with mathematical exactitude and thoroughness because it was the only way I could deliver proof for the influence of zones of interference and disturbance.

Usually it is sufficient for dowsers to concentrate merely on what constitutes a disturbance for a particular client.

The dowsing rod will react at the correct location. It is not always necessary to distinguish between the different kinds of disturbances. The psychologist Ulrich Wiese concurs with me on this point.

Also, it is important to remember that not every disturbance is as harmful for everyone.

Wherever the dowsing rod remains in a neutral (horizontal) position, the client will find a good and undisturbed place.

6. Attitudes of Scientists & Physicians toward Dowsing

(a): Scientists: Otto Prokop, Ph.D., a lecturer at the University of Bonn, says in his book called 'Dowsing Rod, Earth Rays, and Science' (1955), that the turn of the dowsing rod is either fraud or a figment of the imagination.

Also he thinks the dowser belongs either in jail or needs to undergo psychiatric treatment.

It is evident, however, that Dr. Prokop did not familiarize himself with the scientific work done in regard to dowsing before making his accusations.

He also claims that the turning of the dowsing rod could not be reproduced and therefore had no validity scientifically.

I take issue with his position and can support my conclusions with my own scientific work.

Several scientists have countered these accusations. Mr. Oberneder, an engineer proved in his book 'Facts Regarding the Controversy of the Dowsing Rod' (page 6) that already in 1932 the reproducibility of the turning of the dowsing rod was shown in Munich, and that distinguished scientists had already taken a positive stand with regards both to the authenticity of the turning of the dowsing rod and to its value (Dr. Wuest in 1935; Dr. Waither in 1933).

Mr. Oberneder conducted experiments with as many as 450 students, and similar studies were already known from the Dublin physicist Sir William Barrett, and from the radiation researcher Professor Lokofsky of Paris.

Regrettably, Dr. Prokop has misinformed physicians with his book, and even today one still finds adherents of his outdated opinion.

Why is this so ?

Because the majority of physicians are so overworked that they have no time to further their own education.

In addition, the University of Austria has no department of radiesthesia (the study of the sensitivity of humans to earth radiations).

The scientist and physician Dr. Wuest has done pioneering work in this field.

He postulates that rays reach the earth from the cosmos.

Their wavelengths differ greatly, since they vary from nanometers to kilometres.

They are absorbed and reflected to different degrees, depending on the condition of the surface of the earth at a given time and place.

The reflected intensity of the various wavelengths can differ greatly even amongst regions separated by relatively short distances.

He reports on the phenomenon in his book, mentioned above.

He describes how these relationships were measured with highly sensitive portable field intensity apparatus.

Dr. Wuest observed that the small areas of millimetres, centimetres, and decimetres have a marked biological effect which can be felt.

He writes: *"My own observations were correlated by Salzburg's city planner Ludwig Straniak and by French scientist Professor La Varon".*

In a television interview in 1972, Professor Helmuth Hoffman, Ph.D., the Director of the Institute for Electrotechnique, claimed:

"The success of the dowsers is so evident that science can no longer afford to reject them".

The German engineer, Robert Endroes, a specialist in bridge and tunnel construction and a key figure in the construction of the Munich subway, gave a slide lecture at the Austrian Congress for Radiesthesia in 1973. It was entitled 'Structure of the Radiation Field in our Environment'.

He conducted systematic, highly technical experiments and measurements, and came to the conclusion that the global grid has its origin in vibrations of the terrestrial sphere.

At each point of inflection, the shear waves cause a piezoelectric effect which generates an electrical current. This current imposes itself on the crystal lattice of the minerals in the earth.

He further points out that the crossings of the global grid change the field of microwave radiation, and this has an undesirable effect on living organisms.

He also emphasizes that the empirical knowledge assimilated by dowsers over many years in no way conflicts with science.

On the contrary, dowsers with their high sensitivity may pick up influences which escape even highly developed technical devices.

Thus, they often can be the starting point for new scientific discoveries. Mr. Endroes published his findings in the commendable book 'The Radiation of the Earth and Its Influences on Life' (Paffrath Publishing House, Remscheid, Germany).

Professor P. Andreas Resch (Innsbruck-Rome) wrote his doctorial thesis on 'The History and Theory of the Siderian Pendulum, with Reports of My Own Experiments'. This work documents the authenticity of the swinging of the pendulum.

A physicist from l'Ecole Normal Superieur (Paris), Yves Rocard, Ph.D., experimented with ten dowsers who independently looked for and found water at the same locations in a forest, and who also were able to perform experiments in the laboratory with the same degree of accuracy.

There they conducted dowsing experiments within magnetic fields created in the laboratory.

Dr. Rocard assumes that the motion of the pendulum is based on nuclear magnetic resonances.

He observed that the dowsers reacted to extremely weak electromagnetic fields.

The dowsers reported a twitching in the extremities even when exposed to only a few thousandths of an Oersted (unit of the magnetic field strength), of which the dowser was not consciously aware.

The psychologist Ulrich Wiese, MA (Dettelhausen, Germany), gave a paper at the Austrian Congress for Radiesthesia in 1975.

He maintains that a person who is healthy and in tune with his environment will automatically look for the environs in which he can blossom physically, emotionally, and mentally:

"Some zones of disturbance will harm only certain people.; and there are also areas which will be harmful to everyone.

The body of the person who is still healthy will be able to adjust, by avoiding harmful influences and seeking out those from which he will benefit.

In previous times we might have been less susceptible to fields of disturbance, because we might have been more hardy in general."

(b). Practicing Physicians. Several practicing physicians are aware of the value of radiesthesia and use it in their practice. I want to name a few of them.

Arnold Mannlicher, M.D. (Salzburg) wrote in 1949:

"Medical radiesthesia has become of infinite value to me within the past seventeen years.

It has enabled me to achieve diagnostic and therapeutic results which I had never hoped for before".

The chief of pediatric services in Bayreuth, Germany, Karl Beck, M.D., wrote in an article entitled 'Earth Rays' that he observed a patient, released as recovered from the hospital, to become sick again immediately after returning home.

He examined her living quarters with a dowsing rod and found zones of disturbance. When an EKG was administered in her house, she showed extra systolic activity. He examined many people, including dowsers, with the EKG in the years 1956 - 1958.

These experiments showed that sensitive people tend to get sick if they live above a geopathic zone.

The term geopathic, i.e. the illness-producing influence of the earth, was introduced by Professor Walther, M.D., who has conducted many dowsing rod experiments with his students and who has always examined them medically before and after an experiment.

The vegetative nervous system is particularly prone to be harmed, but only after a certain amount of exposure.

However, while the actual dowsing takes place, the reaction to a geopathic zone can be instantaneous.

Thus the average pulse rate of a dowser in Bayreuth rose within seconds from 90 to 200, and then dropped back to 100 after the completion of her work.

The medical director of the Ringberg Clinic, Joseph Issel, M.D., emphasizes in a letter to his medical colleagues:

"Above certain and well-defined areas, the human organism can become seriously affected if he stays there for any length of time.

Eventually he will become ill. A sensitive person can ascertain these areas with the use of a dowsing rod.

We know about so many natural phenomena it is not only our right, but rather our duty to inform our patients of them so as to help them to eliminate or at least avoid their dangers." (A photocopy of this letter is in my possession.)

Ernst Hartmann, M.D. (Eberach) reports about his extensive studies in his book 'Illness as a Problem of Location'.

He made it a routine to examine the sleeping areas of his patients, and especially of those with cancer, with a field-intensity measuring instrument.

He has gained much experience and has amassed convincing material. Again and again he found a correlation between strong geopathic zones and severe organic illness.

Dr. Hartmann also noticed that people who sleep underneath a crack in the ceiling tend to suffer from organic illnesses. He has found that patients improve as soon as they move their bed to another location.

He is convinced that diseases are closely linked to geopathic areas. He writes: *"Usually it takes months or even years before the body becomes sensitized to geopathic irritations it is exposed to.*

Weather fronts are particularly instrumental in provoking physical ailments. The difference lies in the responsiveness of one body type or another".

The C-type (cold type) is highly sensitive to weather influences and to zones of irritation.

Dieter Achoff, M.D. (Wuppertal-Elberfeld, Germany), reported at the Puchburg Congress in 1975 in his paper 'Observations from a Geobiological Practice' that he had achieved astounding results in his medical practice by relocating his patients' beds.

He further states: *"No longer does a physician need great courage to discuss these facts with his patients, since the phenomenon now enjoys general knowledge, due to all the experiments which have been conducted over the years.*

The physician who is cognizant of the existence of zones of disturbance can turn the wheel of destiny to his patients' advantage. For physicians and patients alike the beneficial result is the decisive factor and the justification.

The welfare of our patients is our first and only consideration".

Hilde Plenk, M.D. (Vienna), said in a lecture in the spring of 1977, *"When nothing can be found as the cause of a patient's condition, despite exhaustive tests and hospital procedures, we have to credit the earth rays with being the pathogenic agents.*

This is also true for those cases where finally some 'medical cause' was found, meaning that the geopathic influence had gone on for so long that finally there was organic damage at a demonstrable level."

My own observations corroborate these findings.

Wolfgang Stark, M.D., (Salzburg), who has made many referrals to me, gave me the following explanation in 1975:

"Many aspects of human metabolism depend on bioelectric processes. Electro-physiological studies show that the assimilation of nutrients from the intestines into the lymph and blood stream depend upon a polarization of electrical charges.

On the one side of the cell membrane are plus charges (+); on the other side are negative charges (-).

Nutrients are transported from the intestines into the lymph and blood stream when plus charges are allowed to re-enter the cell.

This polarity will be disturbed in living cells by zones of disturbance".

Dr. Manfred Koehnlechner writes in his thought provoking book 'Nobody Dies in August', on page 156:

"The risk factor associated with one's location needs to be observed much more carefully now than in former times."

7a. What Position Do Physicians and Scientists take in Regard to my Examinations of Living Quarters ?

Since I have become established as a dowser, I have made contact with more than 300 physicians.

While skeptical at first, all of these physicians became impressed with my work - as long as they were willing to take one hour to acquaint themselves with what I was doing !

They became convinced that geopathic influences were indeed at work and that it was possible to establish their presence with the dowsing rod.

During the first few years, I never divulged the names of the physicians or scientists who supported my work and who made use of my talents and skills as a dowser.

I did not want them to suffer the scorn and ridicule of their colleagues, as Dr. Semmelweis had to endure at one time.

But those times have passed, or so it seems to me !

Not only do I think it is justified nowadays, but indeed necessary to identify in this book at least some of the professional people who were willing and open to consider these new possibilities and directions.

And they are no longer in any professional danger !

When I first started my work, I found a zone of disturbance underneath the bed of a well known and very sick woman.

I recommended a change of the bed, and I thought it best to show my diagrams of her living quarters to her physician.

I also wanted to explain the reasons for my recommendation.

I was quite worried as to how to approach the doctor.

However, both he and his wife were most gracious, open minded and genuinely interested.

Consequently, I went into greater detail about my interest in examining the living places of people.

Both of them exclaimed again and again:

"Maybe this patient, or that patient suffers from such influences, since no treatment seems to work."

Finally, this sympathetic and progressive physician, Christian Schaber, M.D., asked me to go with him to visit these patients and examine their bedrooms in particular.

In all seven of these cases, I found zones of disturbance where the bed stood. So Dr. Schaber urged his patients to follow my recommendations and to move the bed to a place free from harmful effects.

After some time, I learned that all seven of these patients experienced considerable relief and that some of them considered themselves cured.

My work started out originally with small children and with children of school age. Lothar R. von Kolitscher, M.D. (Salzburg) asked me to give advice concerning 109 patients, all of whom had responded very little to his long-term efforts.

In every case, I could show zones of disturbance to be present, in many cases there were also Curry and water crossings.

In every case, I sent the exact diagram to the referring physician.

Dr. Kolitscher shared with me that after they followed my recommendation, the patients responded more quickly and with greater success to the medical regime he prescribed.

He also observed that progress was more steady and without the usual ups and downs.

He concluded that the relocation of the bed, that is, the removal of aggravating factors, relieved the patient of considerable physical stress, and allowed them to heal.

This successful doctor said to me on September 9, 1971:

"I thank you so much for your willingness and your devotion, in examining the living quarters of my patients. You really did an outstanding job.

I am not just flattering you, mind you, but I want you to know that you are making a unique contribution to medicine."

That certainly was one of the happiest days of my life !

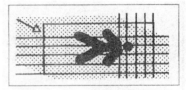

On May 5, 1972, Dr. von Kolitscher said to me: *"You saved this child's life. Only much later will he understand how much he owes you".*

Case# 484b

This eleven year old child had undergone surgery four times because of nodules in the neck area. The complication was that the wound refused to close.

The child's whole body was lying above subterranean water, and his head rested above a Curry crossing.

Only after his sleeping place and his desk in school were moved to a totally undisturbed place, could the medical treatment take effect and the child recuperate.

George Brandstaedter, M.D., said: *"There are many things between heaven and earth that our minds cannot comprehend.*

What counts is that the patient is being helped and especially those patients where traditional medical science is unsuccessful.

Therefore, I will ask you to conduct an examination for my most difficult case." In my presence he called the child's father, and said, *"I have a visitor with me, a dowser.*

Of course, at first I was very skeptical, but after putting her through the ringer, I am convinced that she knows what she is talking about.

There are such things as harmful earth influences and she knows where and how to look for them.

And I would be most interested in finding out whether those influences have something to do with your child's condition.

As you well know, we doctors are at the end of our tether. For years we have only dispensed pain relievers."

I went with the doctor to the house.

The examination established the presence of a wide water current, and also a Curry crossing right where the child slept.

I thought I might be dealing with an anorexic twelve year old, until I learned that the child was already sixteen years old.

Unfortunately, this was one case where the change of bed did not bring quick results.

The family was uncooperative and there was too little understanding and patience. The bed was moved back to the original position and the girl continued to be sick.

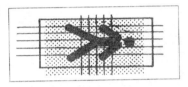

Case# 617

Oswald Poizer, M.D., a general practitioner (Linz, Austria), wrote on January 16, 1974: *"Let me thank you again for all your trouble and caring, and for all the work you went through in giving lectures and writing all those papers.*

You are carrying a light to mankind for the sake of all those who are sick and in need of help."

Franca L. Graf, M.D. (Salzburg) wrote on a postcard on August 19, 1973: *"Your sensitivity and your knowledge will open up new vistas for many sick people."*

The well known physician from Munich, Robert Steidle, M.D., former president of the medical association, reacted with enthusiasm to my lectures and wrote in a letter dated August 5, 1974: *"And when we can help by such simple and harmless measures, does that not constitute true progress ?"*

Karl Kanzian, M.D. (Vienna) told me after my lecture at the Urania:

"Your material is so convincing that ten examples should be enough. And for those who resist what you are telling them, 100 examples would not be more useful."

Hubert Kirschner, M.D. (Tamsweg, Austria), came to one of my lectures and expressed his appreciation for my work afterwards.

Needless to say, the majority of the physicians asked me to examine not only their patients' houses, but their own as well !

They were interested in finding the areas least detrimental to themselves and their families.

A physician for internal medicine, Oswald Ravenelli, M.D. (Innsbruck), said:

"My little daughter used to sleep where you found the water currents. She suffered from constant abdominal pains, and neither my colleagues nor I knew what to do".

In April 1972 I attended a course on 'Autogenic Training', conducted by the Salzburg psychiatrist Kurt Mensburger, M.D.

During the extensive conversation which I had with him afterwards, he said:

"I am absolutely convinced that those zones of disturbance exercise much power.

I have already heard at the University of Salzburg of the work which Dr. Curry has done.

I am personally delighted to have learned so much about it now. From now on, I will advise selected patients to move their bed to another spot in the house."

Ralph Tuerk, a well known German dentist and oral surgeon who had read my book, visited me in 1977.

He invited me to come to his clinic in Bad Pyrmont (Westfalen) and to conduct my examinations there.

He said that he wanted his patients to have the very best chance to get well.

He also arranged for me to give a lecture for physicians and dentists in May of 1978 in Mainz (Germany).

University professors have also had words of appreciation for my work:

Professor Andreas Rett, M.D. (Vienna), invited me to investigate his hospital (Case# 1346). On April 2, 1974, I submitted the results, including the diagrams of all the rooms, complete with notations as to water currents and curry grids.

In my report I made specific recommendations. Professor Rett wrote to me:

"I am personally convinced of the influence of the zones of disturbance. While they are not usually the main cause for the outbreak of illness, they have to be regarded as a contributing factor. We human beings are unfortunately subject to a great many harmful influences.

I thank you, from the bottom of my heart, for everything you did for us, for all your serious work and for your report as well."

Case# 980

Professor Enrico da Silvo-Bastos, M.D. (Sao Paolo, Brazil) said to me:

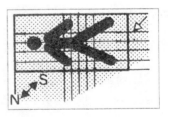

"Your material is convincing, yet I would like to have some personal proof.

We have had a nurse at our clinic for the past six years who falls ill again and again. Even the best treatment does not really work. She wakes up in the morning with severe pains.

I am most anxious to learn if you might find some zones of disturbance underneath the bed of this nurse."

The results of my examination showed both water currents and curry crossings.

Professor Roland Lara Stohmann (La Paz, Bolivia), asked me to examine his own home in addition to his hospital. Since I had to catch a plane, I was unable to examine the hospital, but I was able to examine his house, and there too, his observations coincided with my findings (Case# 938).

Not only did he show great interest in my work, but he also asked me to contact four of his European colleagues. One of them was Professor J. Graz, M.D.

He too, proved to be open-minded and volunteered that from now on, as an experiment, he would recommend a change of bed to those patients who did not respond to his medical efforts.

Professor Andreas Resch, M.D. (Innsbruck) honoured me by calling my illustrations a 'valuable documentation'.

He asked for permission to photograph some of them, so that he could use them in his lectures.

Professor Wilhelm Josef Revers, M.D., the Chairman of the Department of Psychology at Salzburg University (Austria), informed himself thoroughly about my work.

He then asked for an examination of his own home, and finally he approached me to be a lecturer at one of his symposia.

Professor Helmuth Hofman, Ph.D., Director of the Institute of Technology (Vienna), wrote to me after I gave my paper:

"Your material is most impressive. I wish you much success with your work in the future."

Professor Z.V. Harvalik, Ph.D., physicist and the Vice-President of the American Society of Dowsers (Lorton, Virginia), showed great interest in my work.

He wrote to me: *"Your results are convincing and encouraging."*

On one of his European trips he was kind enough to explain to me his own research and its results on 'the biophysical aspects of dowsing'.

To elaborate on the results of these highly scientific investigations would go beyond the scope of this book.

However, the results can be found in the publications of the German Society for Radiesthesia (Issue I, 1974, Issue I, II, IV, 1976, Herold Publishing House, Munich, 71, Kirchbachweg, 16).

A scientific researcher, Egon E. Eckert, an engineer (Newton, USA) published a study entitled 'Sudden and Unexpected Death in Small Children and its Relation to Electro-magnetic Fields'.

He wrote to me:

"I carefully studied your book, 'Discoveries of a Dowser', and I have to tell you that I am very impressed, not only with your skills and with your knowledge, but especially also with the scope of your investigations which have now attained statistical value.

Please accept my sincere wishes for the extensive dissemination of this unique piece of work."

The German engineer, Robert Endroes (Landshut), wrote to me on October 1, 1973:

"I am still very impressed with the lecture you gave in Puchberg.

I was particularly pleased with your thoroughness and the way you explained your observations. My own observations coincide with yours."

Professor Karl Ernst Lotz of the School of Architecture (Biberach) made the following remarks:

"You have done very exacting work. With the technical instruments at my disposal, I was able to confirm the underwater currents at the house of the P. family at exactly the same location that you had indicated in your blueprints."

7b. The Dowser, an Assistant to the Physician

The dowser is not a competitor of the physician, but rather his assistant.

By removing unsuspected obstacles to treatment, he allows the physician to succeed with patients who had previously been unresponsive.

I was a guest in the house of a country doctor. One night, around midnight and during an electrical storm, he was called to the phone.

The very upset parents of a 19 year old girl expressed fear for their daughter's life. She had been lying unconscious in her bed for the past half hour.

They implored the doctor to rush to the house immediately. He went, of course, and was able to save the young woman's life.

He asked me the next day to investigate the young woman's room.

She was lying above water currents and Curry crossings. The bed was moved at once, and within a short time the patient recovered and remained well.

What we need is a rather large number of conscientious, well-trained dowsers who have integrity and who are also willing to dedicate their innate talent to the welfare of their fellow men.

Also, they have to be willing to do their work so as to support the physician. Many people, concerned with the future, and the ever expanding possibilities open to the dowser, share my opinion.

Peter E. Hoch has responded to a need and filled a real void with his book 'Sensitivity to Earth Rays: Primer for the Use of the Pendulum and the Dowsing Rod' (Veritas Publishers, Linz, 1981).

He enlarges on many aspects which are beyond the scope of this book. His book gives an historical account of the development of dowsing, and he addresses himself to the actual work done with the dowsing rod and pendulum. His book constitutes a textbook for dowsers and pendulists.

7c. The Training of a Dowser

Here and there we find a way to do it. I too have trained people without their having had any previous background or schooling. I have done it in groups (Frauenberg/Enns, Munich, Altoetting), but usually in private sessions in many different places, and in many different countries.

The findings of my students always confirm my previous findings and later on they report to me about their experiences.

They and I came to the same conclusions.

Chronically and severely ill people almost always (95% of the time) have their sleeping or working places in areas dominated by water currents and the Curry grid.

Often the two factors are combined, as shown by the illustrations in this book, which represent only a fraction of my 3,000 examinations of houses and apartments.

The areas between the negative zones enjoy helpful and harmonious rays (previously they were called neutral), and those areas are well suited for sleeping and working.

In such areas I found healthy people, almost exclusively.

Because of this practical experience, we urge all dowsers who examine the living places of people to limit themselves to nets, grids, and water currents.

The dowser who merely wants to locate the good places for people to work and sleep should not waste time with considerations of all other factors and possibilities.

This simply consumes too much time, and he runs the risk of appearing a charlatan.

He should stick to what he was trained for: to find the best places for his fellow men to sleep and work.

In order to accomplish this task, it is necessary for him to be exact in delineating the borders of any zone of interference he finds.

It is inappropriate to just give vague indications, since these are likely to upset his clients.

Likewise, since the dowser is asked to find the best possible place, it is not necessary to indicate every area which shows the presence of different geobiological nets, as long as their influence is weak and not detrimental to the client's health.

Under no circumstances should the dowser leave a house or apartment without having shown the 'best place' available. Thus the dowser gives the people a viable choice. Any diagnosis or treatment needs to be reserved for the physician.

7d. Is Dowsing Dangerous for the Practitioner ?

Yes, physically as well as emotionally. Everyone who teaches the art of dowsing needs to be aware of this. He has to point this out to students and teach them how to protect themselves.

Many years ago I was advised by a physician not to train everyone, but only those people who have not only the appropriate sensitivity but also good physical and emotional health.

Furthermore, they need to be people of integrity, with a high degree of self-discipline and thoughtfulness, the kind who use the pendulum or dowsing rod only for the well-being of others and themselves.

Just as the earth is protected by the atmosphere, human beings too, have an invisible protective covering or layer.

However, if people are exposed constantly to damaging rays, as is the case in dowsing, then this natural covering becomes weakened and can no longer protect the person.

Then the dowser becomes physically ill, just as happens to people who sleep or work for years above a geopathic zone.

His heart might function less efficiently, or he might suffer severe emotional damage which might lead to depression or even suicide.

Every profession has its risks. But those who are careful and disciplined will always find new energy to continue their work.

In order to minimize or avoid these dangers, the dowser should put himself into a calm and contemplative state before he sets out on his task.

He needs to maintain health through appropriate diet and living habits. He should not do more work as a dowser than is absolutely necessary.

He should wash his hands under running water after his work.

As a cautionary measure, it is advisable for the dowser to change his clothes and take a shower or bath after exposure to geopathic areas.

He should work as a dowser only when he feels well physically.

He should be cognizant of the weather and avoid dowsing during strong winds, electrical storms or the onset of a cold weather front.

He should see to it that he has sufficient time between dowsing assignments, and if necessary should allow a few days or even weeks before resuming the work.

I know how hard it is to deny our help to ill people who are so anxious for our advice, but these precautions are necessary for the health of the dowser.

The dangers of dowsing are avoided or reduced to a minimum if we search directly for a good place. It is for this reason that I urge all dowsers to use that method.

The dowser should remain standing in the doorway, put himself into a quiet and meditative state, and concentrate on finding the best possible place for his client.

Then he should begin to look slowly in all directions with his dowsing rod extended or with his pendulum hanging down.

As soon as he looks in the right direction, he will feel the pendulum move in that direction or the rod will rotate. The dowser then moves slowly in that direction.

At the centre of this 'good place', the pendulum or dowsing rod will give the appropriate indication. All the dowser then has to do is to find the boundaries of this good place.

After having examined about 1,000 houses and apartments, I was so exhausted that I had to take a long rest.

I met a priest, himself a dowser for 25 years, who suggested that I might use the following prayer before any important work with the dowsing rod or pendulum: ***"May God's will be my will."***

This prayer gave me strength and health so that I could resume my work. At the same time, as my health returned, I recognized that my life work would be the dissemination of knowledge about geopathic influences by giving lectures and by writing this book.

I recommend this prayer to all students of dowsing, as it has brought me peace and strength.

7e. Training of the Dowser with Background in Physics

The exact determination of what points and lines within each disturbed area are apt to produce which particular illness is not something the general practitioner should concern himself with, nor is it within the domain of the 'simple' dowser.

This is a specialized field and should be left entirely to those scientists who have had training in these areas, or to dowsers with special skills.

There has been some speculation lately about 'growth zones', especially on ancient places of worship.

There it was found that water currents and other geological zones constitute a special kind of strong 'stimulus'.

Their influence may well be beneficial for a limited time - several hours perhaps - and may be used at times as a special adjunct to therapy.

But for the long hours of sleep, it is still necessary for a human being to find a quieting place, with harmonious rays.

Much of all this is still in an experimental stage and we have as yet no valid explanation for it.

We have, for instance, no explanation why the Curry grid exercises such a powerful influence.

But many of these as yet inexplicable areas are under investigation by people concerned with the value of dowsing and soon there might be new knowledge arising from their studies.

Scientific investigations of radiesthesia are being conducted by the German physicist Reinhard Schneider (Wertheim).

Everyone who has had the necessary previous training will be most interested in his stimulating course and will profit greatly from it.

He demonstrates that it is possible, depending exactly where a plastic dowsing rod is directed, to distinguish between the various waves, in accordance with physical principles.

Many physicians and scientists have participated in his workshops.

I enjoyed immensely the opportunity to exchange ideas with this knowledgeable dowser on March 7, 1981.

He also liked my book and found it valuable, and he concurred with Dr. Curry that the Curry net was responsible for the development of cancer in certain circumstances.

7f. Empirical Knowledge is Usually Taken Seriously

I never work behind the physician's back.   Rather I attempt to inform as many physicians as possible of the work I am conducting.

I even wrote a short report to the chairman of the Salzburg Society for Preventative Medicine, and also to the president of the Salzburg Medical Association, and I invited all the physicians to my lecture in Salzburg on January 21, 1972.

During the discussion after my lecture, several doctors expressed their agreement with the material I presented, and they clarified some points further.

I was asked to become a member and a collaborator of the Society for Biological and Psychosomatic Medicine in Vienna.

I also spoke about the influences of the earth in a radio interview (Salzburg, Austria, March 1, 1972,).

In September 1972, I sent a short report summarizing my observations and findings based on the examinations of houses and apartments, to the four ministers responsible for the following departments: Art, Education, Health, and Welfare.

As I expected, they too reacted with interest and open-mindedness to my writing.

On July 2, 1975, four Austrian dowsers, myself included, received an official invitation from the Department of Science and Research to come to Vienna and present our work, documents and slides.

There was unanimous agreement at the end that these findings should be made available to other school districts.

On September 15, 1975 I received permission from the Ministry for Education and Art to give guest lectures at the teacher-training academies.

I was particularly pleased when I received an invitation to the Congress for Naturopathy in Freudenstadt, March 1980.

The participants were open and interested, and there was much agreement as to the value of my work.

A group of physicians asked me to give a practical demonstration of how I examine a house.

In this particular house, as in other cases, the subjective 'feelings' of the very sick couple matched with my findings that they were sleeping above a water current and a Curry crossing.

In discussions with these physicians there was much emphasis put on the necessity to include in the diagnosis and treatment of the patients not only the clinical findings, but also the subjective feelings of the sick people.

In the future, remarks such as 'The tests are all negative, therefore it is all psychological', or 'The patient has only a vegetative dystonia', need to be banned from medical usage.

8. Objections and Their Clarifications

I would like to respond to some objections which have been directed to me in personal conversations and in discussions after my lectures.

(a): Some people wonder whether the improvements and the cures which take place after the bed has been moved to a different place might not be due to suggestion only.

While this might be a contributory factor, I think it plays a rather minor role. Otherwise, how can we explain the reactions of plants and animals, and the crawling of infants to a different spot ?

Yet I will not deny that confidence and joyful expectations, even good thoughts, can hasten a cure.

To underline this statement, I quote a letter of August 8, 1973 from a young mother:

"Before we took your advice to move his bed, we had a real sleeping and behaviour problem with our two and a half year old son.

He pressed himself against the bars of his bed, and his arms and little legs would stick out.

The second night after the move he slept through the night for the first time.

Now after ten days there is no more interruption of sleep and he lies stretched out in the middle of his crib".

She also wrote:

"To those who are skeptical, I admit that it might well be possible to influence me by suggestion so that improvement takes place.

But how could a 30 month old child be influenced so that he sleeps through the night ?"

Case# 554

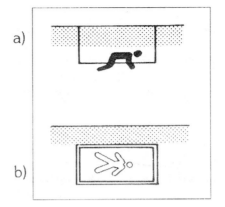

a)

b)

(b). I was asked to comment on the fact that at a certain examination of an apartment, two dowsers made different statements. This was my answer:

"There are also instances where two physicians come up with different diagnoses, and yet we do not reject doctors as a group.

Likewise, we should not reject serious dowsers just because at times they might come up with different results".

A certain physician, who is also a dowser, thought that this is actually inherent in the subject. He gave the following example:

A child, suffering from a very sore throat, is seen by a pediatrician at 11 a.m.

He looks in the child's mouth and sees a severe inflammation, and orders the appropriate medicine.

The pain, however, does not subside, but rather becomes more severe.

The swelling increases and the throat is covered with a white coating. At 4 p.m. the parents summon a specialist to the house.

He has one look at the child's throat, sees the white coating, and pronounces diphtheria.

But five hours earlier, the specialist could not have made that diagnosis either, because the coating was not there.

And at 4 p.m. the pediatrician would also have recognized it.

Likewise, it is entirely possible that a water current runs for only a certain time, so that a dowser can easily find it.

Six months later, another dowser might find no evidence whatsoever for it.

Some water currents carry much water during the winter, while the snow melts, and might be completely dry in the fall.

Therefore, it is important to look for wells in the fall only, when water tends to be scarce.

Also, due to earthquakes or other shocks like blasting or erosion, water currents can change their course.

Nevertheless, I do not exclude the possibility that dowsers and doctors might sometimes make mistakes.

In some cases I have recognized as one of the sources of mistake the fact that the dowser walks too fast.

It is important for the dowser to walk slowly and deliberately and to hold the rod horizontally and taut.

As soon as he feels the turning of the dowsing rod, he has to stop and wait until the rod has turned 90 degrees.

It is of no importance whether the rod turns upward or downward.

In this way, one can delineate exactly the beginning of a zone of disturbance. Only then should the dowser resume walking.

The rod will continue to turn throughout the zone if it is held in such a way that the palm of the dowser's hand is held upwards.

At the end of the zone of disturbance, the rod simply stops turning or swings backward for a short stroke.

If the dowsing rod is held with the palm of the hand downward, then the rod usually remains in the vertical position while the dowser is walking.

At the end of the zone, it positions itself horizontally again.

However, my book is not meant to be a textbook for dowsers, but rather a general source of information.

To people who are interested in, and have a talent for dowsing, I would recommend the book 'Letters of Introduction for Dowsers and Pendulists' by Adolf Flachenegger.

Furthermore, as a basic textbook I would also highly recommend the book by Peter E. Hoch, 'Sensitivity to Rays' (Veritas Verlag). There will always be new discoveries, not only in the medical field, but in radiesthesia as well.

It is therefore very important that the dowser keep up with his field and further his education.

For instance, many dowsers have not yet heard of Dr. Curry's new investigations.

Many countries already have societies for dowsers and pendulists.

The individual dowser should turn to them for training and for access to the pertinent literature.

Indeed, not everyone whose rod does a turn can call himself a dowser. He needs additional theoretical knowledge and extensive experience in the field.

This is of the utmost importance if the dowser is to become a respectable investigator of apartments and houses. He has to be willing to serve, and cannot be driven by monetary considerations.

I would like to point out yet another aspect of dowsing:

Every examination of living quarters takes time and a great deal of energy on the part of the dowser.

Therefore, no one should ask a dowser to investigate his house out of sheer curiosity, but only if he is willing to implement the suggestions of the dowser as soon as possible.

What Socrates said applies here as well, when asking the advice of a physician:

"If someone is seeking health, then question him whether he is willing to avoid the cause of his illness in the future. Only then should you attempt to treat him."

My own findings coincide exactly with those of many successful dowsers.

Often someone says to me:

"Many years ago a dowser told me about water currents at exactly the same spot you have found. But we did not have enough insight then to follow his advice."

(c). During a discussion someone asked me: *"How can you be so sure that water is really under the spot where your dowsing rod makes a turn ? Has anybody drilled for water as a verification ?"*

My answer was *"In the beginning I limited myself to the examination of houses and apartments of relatives and friends.*

I was not sure of myself then. But when I saw again and again how my findings and the complaints of the people in question coincided, their feelings, their pains (being cold all the time, rheumatism, etc.), then I gained certainty and assurance".

Besides, I have to say that many times it has happened that there was subsequent drilling for water.

I quote from a letter from the Tyrolean Bishop, Bonifaz Medersbacher, who now lives in South America (1973):

"A man came from Santa Cruz with an electrical water detector. According to his directions, boring was begun, but very little water was produced.

After that disappointment, the drilling was done at exactly the spot which you had previously indicated, and a very strong stream of water came to the surface, about 4,000 litres per hour.

That meant the salvation for San Miguelito, where in the past it had hardly been possible to get enough water for washing and drinking - let alone to water a garden."

(Note: San Miguelito is an agricultural school in Bolivia, run by Austrian 'Peace Corps' volunteers.)

(d). Someone could not understand how I could spend so much time and energy on such 'superstitions'. This is my reply:

"I consider the examination of people's living quarters not as black magic, but rather as a real help for people. As evidence, I would like to cite the results (Case# 902) of the Bishop Jose C. Rosenhammer of Bolivia.

This bishop grew up in Austria and has served the last forty years not only as the pastor but also 'cultural pioneer' of East Bolivia.

He has been decorated with the highest honours of Austria and Bolivia in recognition of his outstanding social contributions".

Three weeks after my visit to him, while I was still in Bolivia, I received a letter from Bishop Rosenhammer:

" . . and again my heartfelt thanks for your visit and for your help. Considering all the trouble I have had with my eyes over the years, I would never have believed that such a simple repositioning of my bed could bring such dramatic improvements.

I can see how my right eye, which had become very bothersome after surgery, is getting better day by day. . . and if you should get to San Diego, please examine the sleeping place of P. Gottfried who has also had difficulties".

Six months later, another letter arrived: *"... my right eye continues to do well."* (Bishop Rosenhammer had been told that he might become blind.)

I find it necessary to add another important comment: Some religious sects have voiced the opinion that anything beyond direct conscious awareness is 'evil', including the use of the dowsing rod and pendulum.

These statements have caused some confusion, and some dowsers have been thrown into serious internal turmoil.

However, the teaching of the Christian church takes the opposite position. I have discussed this point with many Catholic and Protestant clergymen. Their general consensus is as follows:

"The dowsing rod and pendulum are physical objects, and thus neutral, which means beyond good or evil, as would be a knife or fire or water.

It is true, however, that the misuse of those instruments could become dangerous. But in the hands of people with integrity, who use the pendulum and the dowsing rod only in the service of their fellow men, the effects are most beneficial".

The Swiss Catholic priest Abbe Mermet was given the Pope's blessing for his extraordinary work in dowsing.

The engineer Czepl, a leading Austrian dowser, was invited to the Vatican to assist as a dowser in planning the restoration of the Cathedral of St. Peter.

His task was to determine the path of the subterranean water currents which had severely damaged the walls of the cathedral.

I have several documents which contain positive testimony. One in particular is taken from a letter from a missionary in South Africa, Father Kunibert Reisinger, who has helped many people over the years with his work as a dowser:

"The work with the dowsing rod and pendulum opens new vistas into God's beautiful world, and into the wonders of creation."

I want to add some of my own thoughts to this, and I would like to quote Father Reisinger further:

Let me give you an illustration from my practice: The owner of a large, modern drilling machine asked me for a consultation.

"Father, could you please help me ? Fifteen families, all black, have built their homes nearby. They have collected their money and want to drill a well so that they can obtain drinking water. I don't want to disappoint these people. Please come with me and help me, so that I will be sure to drill at the right spot".

I went with him to the place and began to search with my metal rod.

There was an anthill nearby. Ants build only above water, but who tells them that there is water underneath ?

The creator has given them the sensitivity, the 'feel' for water.

Why should not humans feel for water also ? Drinking water is God's gift.

And should humans be restricted to water only at those spots where it breaks forth into daylight ?

Should we not be able to get water from wherever it can be found, with the aid of technical devices if necessary ?

And again, such devices are based on the laws of nature, with which God has entrusted us.

Thirteen storks arrived in our parsonage in Zululand last week. Who tells these storks that they need to fly south for a few months each year ?

Who tells them where 'south' is ?

They can sense it, for the Lord has given them a special sensitivity to 'south'.

Whenever there happens to be water someplace, it is there whether I know about it or not. And wherever there is no water, I cannot find any either.

I never pick up the pendulum or the dowsing rod without a silent prayer: "Lord, you have bestowed on the bird and the ant the gift of divining. Help me, so that I too, will be able to sense the course of the water, so that these people can obtain their needed drinking water".

Wherever the water is running down there, it creates a certain energy and disturbance. And the sensitive human body is able to ascertain the water's exact location. The dowsing rod in my hands, needless to say, does not find the water. It serves only as a useful tool to indicate to the body where the water can be found.

I found two small currents which were crossing at a certain point. Within eight hours the drill was able to bore a hole twenty five metres deep at the place I specified.

The driller made his first attempt at pumping, and to our delight there was plenty of water spouting forth. Water is a gift from God. And so is being sensitive. Whatever technical device is needed to make this gift available to man is in the end a gift of God also.

(e). Somebody voiced the following opinion: Dowsers, more than other people, have the opportunity to select for themselves a radiation-free environment.

Thus, they should be able to enjoy complete health and well-being.

Otherwise my claim that radiation-free places promote health and well-being will have to be considered wrong and misleading.

My response is as follows: *"Some dowsers are forced to work in places which are not at all free from earth rays. Furthermore, it is not true that we dowsers are able to live a life devoid of radiation. Again and again we have to expose ourselves to harmful rays, and our health is jeopardized every time, and our energies are drained.*

It is therefore important not to request unnecessary work from a dowser, but to limit it to necessary and useful queries".

Prolonged and intensive dowsing can cause severe tension and exhaustion. Therefore, the dowser must see to it that he has breaks so that he can recover from the influences of the radiation.

Many a dowser who did not take care of himself in that way died at too early an age. The dowser can be compared to a pharmacist's scale, which does very useful work, but which cannot be burdened with too much weight.

The Vienna dowser Colonel Beichl worked intensively over many years searching for thermal waters in Vienna.

He sacrificed his life to the research of subterranean radiation. He died of six different types of cancer, although I do not claim in any way that the zones of disturbance were the only illness producing factors.

In conclusion, I want to stress the fact that dowsers have to take particularly good care of themselves. Only then can they be optimally effective in their work.

Smoking, drinking, or excessive eating have all proven to be detrimental to continued effective work in dowsing.

(f). A physician, definitely not without bias and unwilling to inform himself, thought that I should examine a big apartment house, sketch out the zones of disturbance, and only thereafter ask the various people about their state of health.

Only if I could prove a 65% agreement could my work be considered significant.

I could prove to him that I had already done exactly that with as many as twenty-two large houses. The people who lived there told me only afterwards about their health and general condition.

(g). Upset ! Some people voice the opinion that these things should not be discussed since they tend to upset people.

I consider this to be the wrong approach.

We must not hide our heads in the sand in the face of danger.

On the contrary, you may have to commit a small bad act to accomplish a larger good one.

Thus, it is justifiable to smash a window in order to save a person. This opinion was advanced by the Austrian Chief Justice, W. Lotheise (Vienna) in his talk in Bad Ischl in May 1974.

(h). Another physician has argued that my examination of living quarters leads me to engage in unauthorized medical practice.

I am very familiar with the rules governing medical practice and I have never trespassed them. I never diagnosed an illness or gave medical advice.

All I ever did was to ascertain the exact location of the damaging environmental influences in a certain room, and to recommend relocation to a neutral zone.

I made verbatim shorthand records of everything people told me, as something a physician could use in his treatment plan.

In almost all cases I first conducted my examination with the dowsing rod.

It seems rather far fetched to claim that the recommendation to move the bed would constitute interference with medical practice.

Besides, attorneys as well as judges have been to my public lectures and not one of them thought that my work was illegal.

On the contrary, a judge from Salzburg has expressed his appreciation, in a letter dated April 16, 1974, for my work and for my efforts to help the sick.

Thank God we live in a free country in which human rights, freedom of inquiry, freedom of opinion, and the right to pursue serious research are guaranteed.

At this point, I would like to submit a letter from the Chief of Police in Hallein as evidence (Case# 849 from June 13, 1972):

Hallein, May 8, 1974

Dear Ms. Bachler:

I am overjoyed to let you know that your appraisal of my bedroom in regard to water currents and other influences has been a total success. As you know, I have suffered from a nervous heart disorder for the past ten years. As a consequence I felt tired, nervous and lacked interest in anything.

Finally I suffered some sort of collapse, and then my misery was complete. With gratitude I remember the fact that you also advised our daughter to move her bed to another place, as she suffered from exhaustion and nervousness.

My daughter has moved away, and is now free of all those symptoms. My wife and I followed your suggestions and moved our beds.

You told me at the time that I was sleeping with the upper part of my body above a crossing of water and magnetic rays.

A few months after the beds were moved I felt a definite improvement. I can say that nowadays I am completely free of any heart symptoms.

I just wanted you to know this, and also that I support everything you are doing, since your research and your work are doing so much good. With best regards,

George Gastager.

9. Proof for the Existence of Subterranean Influences

(a). We can obtain empirical proof with the aid of mechanical devices, as described on page 18.

There is, however, a simple and somewhat crude experiment, which every person is able to conduct: he can walk through a room with a shortwave apparatus, and at certain points he will hear sounds. Or he can carry a portable television antenna through a room and he will notice certain changes in the picture.

But unsurpassed, at least up to now, is the gifted and experienced dowser with his finely tuned nervous system.

He is able to work with more precision and with greater certainty than any device. For instance, he can tell the depth and the quantity of the water. I remind you of the search for the well in South America.

Goethe remarked:

"The human being himself is the best physical apparatus in existence."

(b). There are also indirect technical determinations possible in regard to the effect of earth influences on humans.

These experiments can be done with the EKG, the EEG, the electro-acupuncture machine, and with electro-magnetic blood tests.

The engineer Professor Kracmar (Vienna), Dr. Beck (Bayreuth), E. Hartmann, M.D., D. Aschoff, M.D., and others have conducted intensive tests.

Their conclusion was that the test results of people above normal soil were different from those obtained when the same people were above 'disturbed' soil.

I too underwent such a test on May 2, 1974. The electro-acupuncture machine was used and my organ values were measured at a neutral place.

Then I was exposed for thirty minutes to the influence of water and Curry crossings and then all the organs were measured again. The values had definitely changed.

(c). There are already several relevant scientific dissertations in existence. I would like to refer briefly to the book by the Swiss hydrologist, Dr. Josef A. Kopp, 'Detrimental Influences of the Earth on Health and on Buildings', (Swiss Publishing House, Zurich).

He claims that above subterranean springs and groundwater currents several abnormal physical conditions will be found, like an increase of the electrical conductivity of the earth, increased ionization of the air, and increased infrared rays. The more elaborate explanations I will leave to the physicists.

I do not consider it within the scope of this book to comment in depth on the papers of these scientists.

Anyone with scientific interest can study the literature himself.

Since I am neither a scientist or a physician, I do not feel qualified to comment on the various investigations done by different experts in the scientific fields. However, as far as empirical evidence is concerned, I am in a position to submit proof for the existence of the 'influences of radiation' without hesitation.

(d). I offer as evidence my investigations of 3,000 apartments and houses - all documented and indexed with date and address, and analyzed in statistical detail.

In those 3,000 examinations I was able to inspect the sleeping areas of about 11,000 people. They fell roughly into the following groups: 1,500 infants and toddlers, 3,000 school-age children and teenagers, and 6,500 adults. Almost all of those records contain sketches.

In the area around the bed I drew in all zones of disturbance.

Those sketches indicate clearly the important factors. In over 1,000 cases, the sketches were drawn with exact proportions.

I see the value of this book in the fact that it can present the evidence to the scientific community and to the public, as well as to physicians and to those who suffer from illness.

I am in a position to prove with a larger number of cases the tendency of plants, animals and babies to avoid zones of disturbance. I consider this to be proof of the influence the earth can exert. For there is no reaction without a previous action.

As further proof, my detailed situational drawings show that people get sick exactly where they are exposed to a zone of disturbance - especially above the intersections of these zones.

The recovery, after the bed has been moved to a place free of radiating factors in the cases of so many people, is the third proof of geopathic influences.

Recovery was measured simply in terms of their just looking so much better and healthier, and also in terms of statements from their physicians and letters written to me.

After recovering, people are often asked by their friends:

"My, you are looking so well, what did you do ?"

Many of these people were previously pale, transparent, run down, tired, exhausted, sad, depressed, discouraged and anorexic.

However, just a few weeks or months after the bed was moved, they appear happy and even exuberant, full of joy for life, with rosy faces and cheeks and shiny eyes - and they had not altered anything else in their lifestyle.

Obviously, I can only cite a few examples in this book. But every scientist and every practicing physician should feel free to inspect my whole collection of factual material.

Since every case is indexed (the number above each drawing), it is possible to find every case at once. It should be understood that every case was recorded truthfully, and that nothing was exaggerated or otherwise distorted. The only changes that were made concerned some of the names, to safeguard confidentiality.

I hope that this book will create enough interest so that more scientists will want to study the phenomenon of dowsing.

And more than anything, I would like to show some of these facts and connections to chronically ill people, so that they can have new hope of finding relief from their illness.

Avoidance of geopathic influences can promise with certainty an improvement in their condition and often even a complete cure.

Of course, many of my experiments were blind tests. I have also recorded several cases of people who, after they felt well again, conducted their own test and moved the bed back to the old place.

Soon they experienced the same problems as before.

Needless to say, as long as my energy lasts I would be most willing to work with any scientist or physician on whatever case they consider interesting or whenever they find themselves at their wit's ends after exhausting the limited resources of conventional medicine.

Repeating an experiment will lead to the same results.

Two years ago I examined a house which was in the process of being built for the W. family. On the plans, I sketched in the water currents as well as the curry crossings exactly to scale, and pencilled in with green colour my recommendation for the location of the beds.

This year I was asked to re-examine the bedroom of Mrs. W. because she suffered from insomnia and from other health problems. The same results were obtained, but Mrs. W. had not followed the instructions conscientiously, and had located her bed thirty centimetres over a water and Curry strip.

10. Ten Indications of the Presence of Pathogenic Zones of Disturbance in the Bedroom.

(Of course, these indicators do not exclude the possible presence of yet other factors.)

1. Aversion to the bed and against going to bed.
2. Not being able to go to sleep for hours.
3. Restless sleep, crumpled up sheet, nightmares, crying out.
4. Avoiding certain spots in the bed, falling out of bed, rocking and head banging.
5. Leaving the bed; 'sleepwalking'.
6. Being cold in bed, shivering, grinding and chattering of teeth; also night sweat.
7. Fatigue and apathy in the morning, often lasting all through the day.
8. Lack of appetite, even vomiting in the morning.
9. Despondency, nervousness, depression, 'just not feeling well', crying after waking in the morning.
10. Cramps, increased heart rate (in bed).

One of these symptoms is enough of an indication; however, there are usually several such symptoms present at one time.

11. How Long before the Relocation of the Bed Brings Relief ?

The change of the location of the bed, or of the place of work, can bring:

(a) Instantaneous Success, and can bring about a complete recovery within a short time, if the zone of disturbance was minimal, and if it was the only negative influence, or if the exposure had taken place only for a short time (not more than two years).

(b) Success can take place soon, after a short time really, often accompanied by reactions due to the change of location.

I always point out the possibility of a location reaction.

To minimize such a crisis I always recommend waiting for a quiet weather front and until an acute illness has somewhat subsided.

This precaution is especially important for heart patients !

In cases of very strong reactions, it is advisable to return the bed to the previous location and to move it gradually, about 20 centimetres per day. I have heard occasionally from adults that they had strong reactions. However, never from children!

E. Hartmann, M.D., wrote: *"Reactions to the change of location constitute a bodily counter-reaction".* He reports of people who, having slept for many years above a zone of interference, experienced reactions the first night, even though their bed might have been moved as little as 50 centimetres.

Occasionally some people moved back to the original sleeping place, because the new one seemed to bring them so much more discomfort.

He further reports that some people ignored his warnings and his recommendations until it was too late.

(c) In some cases, improvement will definitely be slow, whenever there are other negative influences present, or when the patient has taken very strong medication over a period of many years. In that case, the physician might prescribe some measures to detoxify the body and he might try to remove other harmful influences as well.

(d) In some very rare cases, there will be no noticeable improvement. Those will be the cases where the illness has already reached an advanced stage. In such a case one has to be satisfied if there is no worsening of the condition.

12. Did Everyone Report Results after Changing the Bed ?

No, of course not. I do have, however, more than 700 letters so far in which people report to me sometimes a sudden cure and sometimes a slow but steady improvement.

Some people tell me in detail about the improvement they observe in other members of their family. Yet other people write only after many years, when they again need help.

The reason for that may be a new place they moved to or the long illness of a neighbour or friend whom they now ask me to examine on their behalf.

Usually they add something like:

"You helped us so much at the time."

Many people promise to write but procrastinate and finally drop it altogether. Some few people allow themselves to become influenced by the opponents of dowsing.

In the end they claim that the eleventh medication finally did the trick, and that the change in the location of the bed was not important.

Moving the bed back to the original position would prove the correctness of their assumption.

Often I hear indirectly about the benefit people derived from moving the bed, usually from friends whom they refer to me for consultation. And many people are so matter of fact about the whole procedure that they see no reason to inform me.

As an example:

An older man suffered from insomnia, and had experienced two heart attacks.

His physician recommended that I examine the location of his bed.

Water was running underneath the whole length of the bed, and a curry strip crossed diagonally underneath the upper part of the bed.

The bed was immediately moved to a place free of radiation.

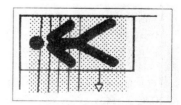

Five months later I inquired into his health.

His answer was:

"Yes, I am really feeling well nowadays.
I moved the bed immediately after you told me to."

He acted as though his success was the most natural thing in the world.

13. Is the Relocation of the Bed Sufficient in
Itself to Bring About a Cure for the Patient ?

No, we need the skills of the physician.

In my public lectures I stress again and again the fact that removal of the bed is not sufficient, but that medical treatment is also imperative.

At the same time, I have also observed in hundreds of cases that the physician could not succeed as long as strong zones of disturbance sabotage his efforts.

In fact, those patients in particular tend to consult many doctors, and each doctor tries to handle the illness with a different drug.

A good physician uses his expertise not only to fight the disease, but also to discover the underlying cause and to eliminate it.

A doctor astute enough to suspect the presence of zones of disturbance is much more effective, of course, and he can bring about a cure in a much shorter time.

Just by asking some relevant questions will he be able to ascertain for himself the presence of zones of disturbance.

He can then recommend that the bed be moved, on a trial basis. Or he can engage the services of an experienced, reliable dowser.

14. Are the Influences from Below the Ground Recognized
by Western Medicine as Illness-Producing Factors ?

Not yet 'officially'. But it will not take very long anymore !

In the 'Standing Room Only' conference room in Bad Reichenhall, I was asked the following question by one of the participants:

"Why were we denied these important facts for the past forty years ? These facts should be told to everyone."

My answer was:

"You are absolutely right. We cannot have sick people waiting another forty years until experts come to some understanding about the physical structure and the effects of these rays. That is why I give so many lectures."

Intuition is always a step ahead of science. Yet science must never negate the facts, but examine them and then find explanations.

I therefore particularly cherish the opportunity to speak before students in the health sciences, and especially to nurses.

And it is for that reason that I make a special point to contact university professors so that I can acquaint them with the facts concerning the influences within the earth.

I hope that soon this whole range of ideas will be taught at the universities.

I have had many opportunities to speak during conferences and meetings with leading scientists, especially with physicians.

I was able to give them a brief exposé about the workings of the zones of interference within the earth.

I mention this only because some physicians are still afraid of what their colleagues will think of them if they admit their interest in these phenomena.

I very much want to encourage those physicians to familiarize themselves with these important facts.

A television show in Austria on April 28, 1977, gave a very objective report about my research in schools, as well as about my many lectures.

At the end of the programme, the very courageous producer of that show, Mr. Elmer Oberhauser, interviewed Dr. Johann Kugler, one of the most progressive professors of medicine at the psychiatric hospital in Munich, Germany. He said:

"There is meteorological evidence for fluctuations in the earth's magnetic field. Certain disturbances in the magnetic field above subterranean water currents can cause illness in people. That has been proven without a doubt, and can be verified with psychological testing methods and with reaction time tests."

A television show in Austria on April 28, 1977, gave a very objective report about my research in schools, as well as about my many lectures.

In my many discussions with physicians I have realized that it is not always just pride, arrogance, lack of interest or unwillingness - as many people maintain - when physicians reject the insights and evidence of dowsers and pendulists.

There are some real problems. For nothing like this has ever been taught at the university.

Some consider the whole approach too simplistic; others have met up with charlatans.

Lately, however, there has emerged a real willingness and readiness. Traditional medicine, too, has recognized that not only compassion, but also fairness in regard to their patients, makes it imperative that they seek out the underlying causes of an illness.

Many well established physicians speak out on radio and on television and state that they welcome the occasions when causes of a disease are brought to their attention - causes of which they had not known up to that time.

Many of them have already started to educate themselves seriously about the phenomenon of dowsing, and to integrate this knowledge and skill as a useful tool into their practice.

In practical terms it means that they recommend the relocation of the patient's bed in chronic cases, or for those who suffer insomnia. This fact has been brought to my attention again and again by readers of my book.

Another step which points to the increasing openness of traditional medicine is the fact that I have been invited more and more frequently to meetings for physicians, not only as a participant, but as a lecturer and discussant as well.

15. Auras and Kirlian Photography

Dr. Karl von Reichenbach (Austria) recognized that every human being possess a 'radiation body', which he first called the 'Od' and later the 'aura'.

He did his first research in Vienna and wrote the famous 'Science of the Od'.

Some particularly sensitive people are able to see the aura. The Russian research couple, the Kirlians, made the aura visible to everyone by means of high frequency waves and preserved the image by photographic processes.

They called this phenomenon the 'bioplasma body'. This bioplasma body envelops the firm, physical 'bioelectrical' body like a cloak with many different lights, like a beautiful and mysterious firework display.

Animals and plants, as well as humans, possess a bioplasma body.

The Kirlians advanced the theory that human beings receive external radiation first with their semi-material bioplasma body and that it is then conducted to the vegetative nervous system.

The Austrian physician Heinrick Huber (Vienna) said in his lecture, 'The Life Force in Man', in Puchberg (1975):

"The energy body (radiation body) will manifest illnesses before the physical body does. The life energy is guaranteed through the breath. The breath renews it, maintains it, and influences our physical being."

What factors influence our bioelectrical energy field ?

- Natural energy fields (earth, cosmic);
- Artificial energy fields produced by artificial devices (electricity, television, radio, etc.);
- Energy fields generated by those around us, especially with their various emotions.
- Goodwill, love, joy, confidence and trust will have a strengthening influence.

Unfriendliness and distrust hold us back and produce negative and defensive attitudes in us. Parents and educators should always be aware of this.

People cannot be turned on and off like machines (and some people are particularly sensitive), but the attitude of those around them plays a decisive role.

For instance, the attitude of those who watch a dowser at work can either have an energizing effect or a debilitating effect.

16. Depth, Quantity and Direction of the Water

It has been observed that deep running water does not have a lesser effect, but rather a stronger one, than surface water.

It has also been observed that rays can be felt just as strongly on the highest floors of a skyscraper.

Also of importance is the direction in which the water runs, the quantity of water, the angle at which it runs, and its speed.

It has also been shown that the edges or borders of the flow, even in subterranean waters, are very influential.

This can be compared to streams above ground, where banks may suffer especially from erosion.

Adolf Flachenegger observed during his 50 years of activity with innumerable cases, that 'pushing waters', that is, waters which run in the direction of the feet to the head, can cause congestion of blood in the head, nightmares and depressions, often leading to suicide.

These claims were at first unacceptable to Professor Kracmar (Vienna), a scientist who then concentrated his investigations on this particular aspect and found that it was indeed the case.

At a meeting in Puchberg in 1973, he explained these facts in great detail in his paper 'Scientific Reflections about the Bio-logical Effects of Pushing Waters'.

Eleven papers given at this meeting in Puchberg can be found at the Society for Dowsing (Vienna), and are available for inspection.

Like Flachenegger, I have been able to recognize the effect of 'pushing waters' in very many cases.

We further observed that the 'pulling waters' - running from the head to the feet - can cause dizziness, blacking out, loss of balance, and even fainting.

The latter will happen only if in addition to strongly pulling water there is also a strong crossing of zones of disturbance.

In my case histories I will give several such examples.

17. Can Traffic Accidents be Caused by Earth Rays ?

Yes, we have already collected much material on this subject, based on observations and investigations from many countries, especially Austria, Germany, the USA, and Switzerland.

In addition to the pioneering work done by Arnold Flachenegger, Egon Sarcilly-Ernes, an engineer from Vienna, has devoted much time and energy to this subject.

Thanks to his efforts, lectures, and personal engagements, he has been able to awaken the interest and understanding of some influential officials in Vienna.

Finally he was given permission to train a few selected policemen in the art of dowsing.

At the Congress for Dowsers in Puchberg (Wels), September 11, 1977, a slide lecture was delivered by Robert Endroes, a German scientist (Landshut), about his newest and most interesting results, 'Head on Collisions Caused by Subterranean Waters'.

He also had found some plausible scientific explanations for the 'blocking' of the driver's concentration.

All those infamous spots in the road where frequent terrible accidents happen 'without any obvious reasons' are located in severely disturbed zones of underground interference.

Some countries have put warning signals with speed limits at those particular points.

18. Is There a Way to Counteract or Screen Out Earth Rays ?

Of course, there are some researchers who are concentrating on finding a way to render these disturbance zones harmless. There is even some neutralizing equipment on the market.

However, this is still very expensive, and only effective for a very limited time. It is also very difficult to install, and if not done correctly, it is totally useless.

Dr. Issels, M.D., stresses in his letter to physicians (cited earlier) that *"to neutralize the effect of earth radiation with technical devices is still problematical. In principle, we always recommend the relocation of the bed, or a change of the apartment or house".*

I too recommend that the bed be put in a different place.

I find that this is almost always possible, although people are sometimes reluctant at first. If worst comes to worst, one can fasten wheels on the bed and roll it to a good place at night, for instance in the middle of the room.

This advice worked instantly for Mr. and Mrs. Haugler (Case# 1922). He wrote: *"...and since then we feel as though we have been rescued to an island."*

There are now investigations in progress which are based on a transformation of energy and which therefore promise to be effective as far as the neutralizing possibility is concerned. However, I am not familiar with this work.

Furthermore, it would be impossible for me to re-examine the living spaces again in all the different countries. This would be necessary in many of the cases so that the neutralizers could be positioned accurately.

Therefore, I wrote to all those who have approached me. I asked them to re-read carefully the last chapter in my book and to follow the recommendations I have given.

In all probability, they can take care of their problems themselves, and will not need the service of a dowser or the aid of a neutralizing device.

19. Are There Other Environmental Influences
to Which We Should Give Attention ?

(a) The environmentalists ask us to reflect on certain aspects of our lifestyle. They help us by providing us with information.

In general, we need to pay attention again to a more healthful way of living, to better nutrition, to sufficient sleep (particularly before midnight), to better breathing, to outdoor exercise, and to the use of natural materials in our clothing, bedding and furniture.

Most people have adverse reactions to iron and synthetic fibres.

Therefore, it is better to have a wooden bed frame, mattresses from natural fibres such as wool, cotton or seagrass, and to use a wooden chair instead of an iron swivel chair.

I also want to mention that a steel wristwatch and a watch with a radioactive face can be definitely detrimental to people's health.

The electric current of household electrical circuits can be a great source of irritation. Many doctors have come to the conclusion that in our day and age, not only the earth rays, but also the artificial rays from radios, television, and electrical appliances are increasingly responsible for disturbances in sleep patterns, for headaches, lack of enthusiasm for living, and depressions which often lead to suicide.

Many people cannot free themselves from the feeling that they 'cannot stand it anymore'. Some people react to this 'artificial stress' by becoming hostile, aggressive, and in general difficult.

This is especially so when they also sleep over a 'disturbance crossing'.

One must see to it that there is no electrical appliance like a refrigerator, freezer, television or radio next to one's bed.

Such appliances should also not be situated behind a wall next to the bed, because their rays penetrate the wall. The minimum distance should be two metres.

That also goes for tape recorders and electric or battery-run alarm clocks, and lamps on a nightstand or over the bed should be at least 75 cm (30 inches) removed from the body.

Neon lighting above the head is also detrimental to one's well-being. I have seen several cases where the bed was put next to the wall, on the other side of which stood a television set.

From that time on, the people suffered from severe headaches, insomnia and depression. The children, from that time on, would not stay in bed anymore. This negative influence is at work even though the set might not be turned on at the time. And when it is turned on, we find that the influence is more intense, and that it penetrates several metres right through the walls !

We need to be mindful of our fellow men !

The television set should always be put behind a wall adjacent to a hallway, or on an outside wall.

Professor Herbert Koenig (Munich) published his results based on many years of research on the effects of electricity in his book 'Invisible Surroundings'. He points out that we are surrounded by electromagnetic forces (expressed in our sensitivity to weather and field intensity and in effects on the dowsing rod).

Dr. Werner Kaufmann (Atzbach) has been an expert in environmental studies for years. Walter Kumpe, environmentalist and architectural biologist, wrote a very interesting little book in which he gave an overall view of the pertinent problem 'Are Our Houses Making Us Sick ?' (Paffrath Press, Remscheid).

Among other things, he points out that there is some acknowledgement of these important connections, since biologists and technologists in the field of 'bionics' are beginning to work together.

(b) Biologists concerned with the environmental impact of our houses and living quarters on our health and well-being are also pointing out very pertinent problems.

Professor Anton Schneider, known to be a responsible scientist, was looking to the future when in 1980 he founded the Institute for Building Biology (Rosenheim).

This institute offers a well-rounded 'building biology' training for architects and contractors; he also publishes the magazine 'Healthful Residences'.

Anyone who wants to build a house would do well to seek information and to acquaint himself with the problems long in advance. Professor Schneider invited me to collaborate with him (Publication No. 4).

Professor Karl Ernst Lotz, a chemist, offers a primer, 'Buildings and Residences', which has proven to be very helpful for many people.

The architect M. Mettler and the builder H. von Gunten invited me to work with them as a dowser in Switzerland.

We agree in many aspects of our work, for example, on the importance of the Curry net.

And many other architects, builders and contractors have told me that they now have building lots examined for water currents and other disturbances before breaking ground.

My book convinced them of the importance of geobiological effects.

They have also recognized the value of natural, non-synthetic building materials, since people report much greater enjoyment from living in houses built that way.

It is important to strive for harmony in all aspects of our lives, and that includes the way we build our homes.

20. Handling Everyday Living with Ease

A woman from Vienna wrote me after she had moved her bed:

"It will please you to hear that I no longer wake up in he mornings as though I had spent the night in a nightmare, that I am no longer lethargic and tired, and that I no longer expect the day to be just too much to get through ... I cannot tell you how happy I am."

The letter of a very busy young mother contains the following paragraph:

"Soon after we relocated the bed I began to sleep deeply and without disturbance, and very soon I began to feel so much better in general.

During my period, too, I no longer have headaches, the depressions are gone, no more cramps and no more pain.

I am also not so tired anymore and now I can handle my daily tasks with ease."

21. Pride and Indecision preventing a Necessary Change

Mr. Franz. N. requested an examination of his apartment. After I gave him my recommendations, he had a difficult time making the necessary alterations. He tells about this in an extensive letter, which I would like to quote in its entirety.

Salzburg, September 29, 1974.

Dear Ms. Bachler,

Please excuse my responding after so much delay concerning your recommendations about our bedroom.

This has been a hectic time for me, but I also have to confess to a certain personal indifference, once the desired results were obtained. I simply procrastinated in letting you know about the effects of the changes you recommended.

Once again, I trust you will accept my apologies.

Let me tell you what happened when we finally did what you had suggested. Before anything else, I want you to know that my wife and I are extremely grateful to you.

For almost instantaneously, we felt a great deal better than before, and the culmination was that we are now free of the ailments which had given us trouble for such a long time.

We did not tell you at the time that my wife had such severe pain in her arm that it was almost impossible for her to touch anything with her left hand. Extensive medical treatment gave no relief.

I myself suffered from such debilitating insomnia that I often felt as though I could not go on. You might remember that we had a built-in wardrobe in the bedroom, and that the rest of the furniture too, was put in what seemed to be the only logical place.

And when you announced that it was imperative that we change things around according to your specifications, I panicked a bit, since I could not imagine how this would work, even though I have some experience as far as planning is concerned.

It may have been my pride also, since I had spent much time, energy and thought on redoing our bedroom. And we had had it completed just a short time before.

Perhaps you can understand how difficult it seemed for me to submit to your recommendations. Even when you said goodbye to us, I felt reluctant to pay attention to what you had said.

However, you had said one thing to my wife, which repeatedly came up for me.

You told her that sooner or later she would have trouble with her arm if she did not already have some. I picked that up, since we had not mentioned anything about that to you and since there were no signs you could have observed.

On the same evening, we began to contemplate what would be involved in carrying out your recommendations, and I buried myself in the plans.

We started to measure and re-measure, always remembering your recommendations, and lo and behold, suddenly the whole idea no longer seemed absurd.

Certainly, some things had to be shifted around and had to be redone, like new electrical outlets etc., but that did not seem to be such a big obstacle anymore. We began with the re-modeling the following day, and before we knew it, everything was completed.

The first night I immediately slept so much better. I thought it was a coincidence, since I was very tired from working so hard physically that day. No way would I have credited you and your recommendations with the success.

Case# 1407

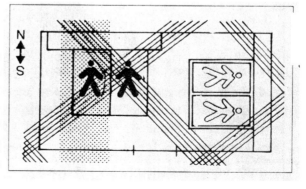

However, I began to sleep well every night, and finally I had to admit that the relocation of the bed had brought about this beneficial change.

I also noticed that my wife was no longer supporting her hand.

She became aware that her condition had improved only after I asked her.

Today she is absolutely sure about it and she has no pain at all anymore.

Thus we owe you much, dear Ms. Bachler, because without you we would never have thought of doing this.

Enclosed you will find a sketch of the original and the present living arrangement. If your time would permit it, we would be so happy to show off the new room to you.

  With best regards, gratefully, your family N.

22. *"That's Simply Incredible !"*

That is what many people exclaim when I tell them about these facts and connections. Yes, I really believe that they cannot comprehend it, especially since the truth is so simple.

They have built a logical system, and this system might now collapse. The words of a wise person come to mind who said, *"He who can never retract an opinion loves himself more than the truth."* And the poet, Mathias Claudius, expresses these thoughts in his much beloved poem:

  Do you see the moon up there?
  Only half of it is visible
  And yet it is round and splendid
  And so are many things
  At which we just laugh
  Since our eyes cannot perceive them whole.

This poem, which is often sung as an evening song, reminds me of my father. He sang many happy songs to us, songs and poems which mirrored a deep faith, a loving sense of humour, and a deep relationship to nature.

This attitude helped my parents overcome the troubles they suffered from the zones of disturbance over which they lived.

Of course, they had no idea of their existence.

I had a happy childhood. I was surrounded by loving parents and siblings.

The memories of meadows in bloom, the fragrance of the hay, the forest, and the fields are unforgettable for me, as is the way my father walked, slowly, deliberately sowing seeds.

And the ripeness of the grain, the sunshine and the shimmering stars at night, the singing of the birds, the crystal clear brooks, the mountains and the drifting clouds...

Only one thing cast a shadow over my happiness: our dear mother was sick most of the time. Now I am certain that this was caused by a crossing of zones of disturbance.

I remember how much I pitied my mother, even when I was only four years old, when she complained just after going to bed:

"Now my feet are cramping up again."

And then at night she could not sleep for hours because of so much pain. Sometimes she would literally flee from her bed for several hours.

When she was first married, she was so ill that she had to go to the hospital.

At last her body found an equilibrium and renewed its vitality.

This did not happen by regular, sound sleep, but rather during the day through physical work outdoors.

Her faith and her belief in prayer helped her, as did her love for her children and her feeling of responsibility before God.

She was able to get through life for 50 years sustained by her faith.

And she also experienced what so many sensitive people have to go through: she was misunderstood, even by us children at times, when she complained about tension, depression and even pain, 'without any reason', often two days before there was a change in the weather. But our father was always good to her.

The illness of my siblings and me put a damper on our happiness. Here again, the ultimate factor was the zones of disturbance.

As a child I suffered from stomach aches, nausea and vomiting. I learned to live with it. Now I know that I was born with a gall bladder defect, which was the cause of much of my discomfort.

I am sure that this abnormality, in addition to an innate sensitivity, accounts for my greatly developed sensitivity to rays.

Strong tension over zones of disturbance frequently activates the old gall bladder, liver and intestine troubles.

My life has been in danger three times.

Once when I was very small, again at the age of 36 years after I had been lying above a curry-water crossing for seven years, and finally a few years ago - after I had examined more than 1,000 geopathic residences within a very short time.

Dr. Lothar Kolitscher saved my life, and I will be forever grateful to him.

Yet, I had a very hard time saying NO to the urgent requests for help from so many sick people.

But then I recognized that often a change of the location of the bed just 'for better or worse' could be of great help.

I was not allowed to work with the dowsing rod for more than a year.

Finally, it became clear to me that my main task consisted of spreading the knowledge about the zones of disturbances in lectures, informal talks, and in the form of this book.

Also, I had to become much more careful about how much practical work I was willing to do.

I am now well aware of these relationships, and am able to avoid zones of interference in my own apartment.

Therefore, I am in much better physical condition than ever before.

Of course, I am taking care of myself in other respects also.

There are chronically ill people sleeping over zones of disturbance in every country, in every city and village.

Many do not know any better, but in some cases, it is out of false pride that they reject as 'nonsense' these old traditions which are preserved in folklore.

At this point, the last verse of the 'Evensong' comes to my mind, in which the poet tells us:

> Lie down to sleep, brethren,
> In the name of the Lord.
> The evening breeze is cold.
> Do not punish us, oh Lord
> But let us sleep in peace
> And grant our ailing neighbours
> A restful night, as well.

We dowsers are grateful to be allowed assist.

Käthe Bachler

Part II - FAILURES IN SCHOOL
POSSIBLY CAUSED BY GEOPATHIC ZONES
OF DISTURBANCE AT HOME AND IN SCHOOL

1. Zones of Disturbance and the Educational System

Is it surprising that those children whose sleep is negatively affected by radiation exhibit behaviour as though they were lazy ?

They are tired, listless, their concentration span is short, and their work in school is frequently inadequate.

The very timid ones, the slowpokes, the sleepyheads, those who were labeled as 'lazy', the forgetful ones, those who seemed to play truant, the hyperactive ones, and the ones who were just difficult to handle in my class - those were the children who were damaged by zones of disturbance.

As soon as I recognized what it was all about, I considered it my duty to explain to these children the reasons for their failure and to assist them in removing those influences.

Thus I could help them to perform better. As a classroom teacher, I had plenty of opportunity to do this.

In a lecture 'Zones of Disturbance and the Educational System', given at the Austrian Congress for Radiesthesia in 1973 in Puchberg (Wels), I reported some of my findings in great detail and illustrated them with slides.

I would like to begin the discussion in this book about school failures by writing about an experience I had.

Ursula, a Concern for Parents and Teachers

Many years ago Ursula was my student. Her intelligent parents were amazed and could not come up with any explanation why this child behaved so differently from her brothers and sisters.

She was always moody and very difficult to handle. Despite her intelligence, she practically failed in school. Ursula paid no attention in class.

She was disruptive, stubborn, aggressive, and her performance was poor.

Later on, when Ursula left home, she began to feel better. Her self-esteem increased and she became successful.

She is now appreciated and liked by all who meet her.

A few years ago I was asked by Ursula's parents to examine their residence. In one of the rooms I found a Curry crossing right above a water current.

Both parents exclaimed simultaneously, *"This is exactly the spot where Ursula's bed stood from junior high school on!*

We all were very upset and sorry that we had not known the cause of her difficulties at that time.

We had thought that we were dealing with laziness, sloppiness, and weak character, and that it was all her own fault.

Instead we realized that night after night the strength and vitality of the child was simply being drained away."

On that occasion I also learned that Ursula suffered from terrible nightmares almost nightly.

She would toss and turn half the night and scratch incessantly.

No wonder she was tired and depressed all day.

We later talked with Ursula about all of these things.

Some readers might want to think back on their own childhood, and recall whether they felt similar to Ursula.

In doing so the reader should keep in mind that neither parents nor teachers could be omniscient, and that in retrospect they would probably regret the fact that they did not know about geopathic disturbances at the time.

They could only judge on the basis of the behaviour shown to them. Ultimately, parents as well as teachers want the best for children.

The reader might also keep in mind that in many cases parents and teachers, because of their own exposure to earth radiation, are at the end of their tether.

That was definitely true for me for many years.

I had no inkling of all the things I have learned in the meantime.

At least now I am able to help people, including my students, because of my own experiences.

I am happy and grateful for that.

2. Pre-School Age

It is important to include the pre-school age in our considerations, since we also know that poor school performance often results from damage suffered in early childhood years.

1. The influence of the zones of disturbance on beings in utero.

When such zones cause tension and illness for the mother, this can indirectly lead to organic defects and even malformations in the foetus.

The zones can directly affect the foetus, causing defects, weakness, or toxicity.

I followed many cases like that.

We also frequently find that the influence of the zones is the cause of premature birth or spontaneous abortion.

These facts have not yet been taken seriously enough. I refer to case# 610.

2. The consequences of a long and difficult labour and delivery for the later development of a child has been generally recognized.

It is well known that tension in the mother can provoke a difficult delivery and possible brain damage, not even recognized by the parents, can lead to learning disabilities later on.

Little attention is paid, however, to the fact that susceptible women, who are lying over a zone of disturbance during labour and delivery, may suffer great tension and even convulsions.

Thus, the zones of disturbance can be the culprit at the time of birth, too.

Therefore, it is particularly important to provide a woman with a place free of radiation during her pregnancy and delivery.

In Part I, Section 3, entitled 'How Do Humans React to Subterranean Water Currents ?' I explained that infants and young children instinctively flee from radiated areas.

I also mentioned that babies and small children, who are incapable of avoiding those areas by themselves, might suffer severe damage if they are confined to their cribs, despite their cries and screams of protest.

My proof is the material I have collected on 1,500 babies and small children. I have included fifteen examples in the case-study section of this book.

It seems evident that damages which were caused by zones of disturbance, such as slow development, stuttering, convulsive crying or screaming, or serious illnesses like meningitis, convulsions or even unconsciousness in early childhood, can be an inhibiting factor in normal intellectual development and thus often the reason for school failure later on.

Even in school entrance exams we can see the consequences of these detrimental effects.

3. School Age

My observations about this very specialized field of dowsing are based on the examination of apartments and houses of 3,000 pupils and students.

So that parents and teachers can convince themselves of the effect of the zones of disturbance on children of school age, I will cite 40 examples as illustrations.

Success in school is dependent on many factors: innate ability, physical and emotional well-being, education and training, willingness to apply oneself, etc.

Likewise, school failures are also dependent on many different factors. But one of the real causes is often the presence of zones of disturbance.

So far we have not given these factors enough credence. An intelligent child is normally curious, eager to learn, and willing to please.

If he fails in school despite all of these attributes, then parents and teachers alike are puzzled and cannot come up with any explanation.

1. The reaction of a child to a zone of disturbance can be very different, depending on the kind and strength of the zone, and also depending on the constitution of the person:
- depending on whether we have a robust or sensitive child,
- depending on whether the child is well or already ill,
- depending on the kind of influence,
- depending on the weather conditions,
- depending on whether we have to deal with the zone of disturbance by itself, or whether other harmful factors are present.

Water by itself usually causes fatigue and lethargy. Curry crossings, however, bring about restlessness and nervousness.

Another factor is whether the child is exposed to only one area, like his bed or his desk at school or his place to do homework at home, or whether he is exposed to two or even three of these crossings of zones of disturbance.

In the former case we may see that the work in school is not commensurate with the child's innate ability; in the second case we will see that the child suffers from ill health within a short time and that he may fail in school altogether.

2. The student's bed was above strong zones of disturbance:

a. Very nervous children (Case# 658, p.135; #984, p.133), fidgety and agitated, who give up easily and don't dare even try, who have trouble making contact with others, whose self-esteem is low and who cry easily.

Some of these children wake up in the morning with fear and dread of the day ahead.

b. The slowest (Case# 265, p.137) the dawdlers, the always tired ones.

No wonder, for they could not get to sleep the night before for many hours, and even after that their sleep was restless.

They felt nauseous and could not get their breakfast down, and some of them retched afterwards. Nature forced some of them to make up for lost sleep during school hours.

c. Those who appeared lazy (Case# 153, p.138) because they sat listlessly in the classroom, and often had not done their homework.

But what really went unnoticed was that they were very tired, their energy level was low, and they could not concentrate on their school work.

Thus they could not master their work. Some of them tried to lie their way out of the threatened punishments. They were in a perpetual state of fear.

Some of these children had to stay after school many an afternoon, and they were always reprimanded for not applying themselves better.

d. Those children who were forgetful. Their forgetfulness was taken as a character flaw. Through reprimands, threats, and punishment, the parents and teachers tried to 'help the memory along', usually without success.

What was really going on was a lack of thinking and remembering ability because of the noxious zones of disturbance.

But since the children usually did not know any more about those causes than did their parents or teachers, the children themselves believed after a period of time that they were indeed lazy and careless, and deserved to he punished.

They suffered from guilt feelings all the time. They had the best of intentions and promised to do better, but did not have the energy to carry it out.

How much suffering some people have to go through, even in their early years of life !

e. Children who played truant (Case# 162, p.140). Some of those students who suffered for what seemed a long time through the hopeless situation of severe fatigue, failure and punishment, finally tried to escape this vicious circle by staying away from school with some kind of flimsy excuse.

They simply could not cope with the work any longer. There were by now too many incompletes in their work. They felt unable to follow the instructions, and finally just capitulated. Then they were labelled truants.

What really went on was that they were so weakened by their nightly battles (with dizziness, tightness in the chest, nausea and vomiting), that they were unable to go to school in the morning.

f. The most restless and the most difficult ones. Many of them were always in a bad mood, aggressive, hostile, impertinent, and anti-social.

The other children teased them at first, and finally avoided them altogether. The teachers punished them, which they felt was unfair.

It is in this connection that I would like to ask your indulgence and be allowed to make some pedagogical comments.

Cynicism and sarcasm, when used without love, must be considered education's true enemies. Not only should parents and teachers never use them, but they should also see to it that children never use them amongst themselves.

Rather parents and teachers should appeal to the good sense of a child and make an attempt to eliminate the cause of whatever the problem seems to be.

They need to help and also educate children to be helpful to each other.

Nothing is harder to tolerate than constant needling. Having been taunted for a long time, or having been exposed to verbal insults can result in physical illness for some people. Psyche and body cannot be separated.

Even children may suffer from emotional rigidity and from such strong defenses that they need to be helped to soften them.

More and more I recognize the wisdom of Marga Mueller (Munich) in stressing the importance of human interaction based on appreciation and praise, on asking and thanking, on recognizing and acknowledging wrongdoing, on asking to be forgiven and on making amends.

These basic forms of human interactions are necessary for harmonious living within a family, in schools, communities, states and finally in the way various countries work out their differences.

They are the essential foundation for the relation of man to God.

I think with great respect and gratitude of my own parents and teachers who have taught me those fundamental forms of human interactions.

The training for courage and fortitude needs to start early in life.

The fear of other people, the fear of being ridiculed or thought a fool, are among the great hindrances in life.

This is true in the life of adults as well, not just children. A motto can serve as a great help, and I am reminded of the words of Don Boscos.

He was a benefactor of thousands of young people and let his life be guided by this one sentence:

"The best we can do in this world is to serve others,

be joyful, and let the sparrows be as they are."

We all know that love exercises the greatest influence in the educational process, both the love we receive and the love we give. Julius Langbehn expresses this thought in the following way:

"Fruit ripens in the warmth of the sun,

Human beings flourish in the radiance of love."

Some young person struggling with his own self-preoccupation and wanting to open up to others might be helped by the following:

"And this is your purpose in the world,

That your being will make it brighter."

Maybe some of these thoughts will serve as encouragement for a young teacher, embarking on his or her life work.

For I am absolutely certain - and it is an ill-founded reproach that I am only interested in eliminating the zones of disturbance - that an education based on human values is a great help for any child's success in school and for a happy life later on.

Whenever children ask me to write something in their scrapbook, I do not treat that request as 'just one more thing to do', but rather as an opportunity to give them a motto or an aphorism that could accompany them through life.

While writing I always concentrate with good thoughts and feelings on that particular child.

I myself am convinced of the power of positive thinking.

Every good thought, every good deed, is like a pebble cast upon a lake. This pebble produces waves which expand and expand.

Unfortunately, the same happens with our negative thoughts and our careless words.

That too, is something children need to hear about.

The following poem was my most frequent selection to write in their album, scrapbook, or just on a nice card:

> *"Good I will be and I will make others happy,*
> *And I will turn suffering into joy and laughter.*
> *I want to bring warmth and comfort to many*
> *So that my very being is but a blessing."*

Sometimes I hear many years later from these people that they still read that poem from time to time.

Poems like this, given to children as a guide, can play a great role in our intellectualized life for awakening emotional and spiritual value.

At the same time it is important for us as parents, teachers and educators not to force children, and especially not adolescents (or even our fellow adults), to 'do good' but rather to gently invite and encourage them.

We need to be an example upon which they can model themselves.

An educator expressed this attitude as follows: *"The good shepherd does not go behind wielding his stick, but rather in front, gently coaxing".*

We also need to be careful not to treat all children alike.

We need to see each child in its environment, with its own talents and personality and its own individual nature.

Only if the child is appreciated within his own framework is he willing and able to do his very best.

When the child feels that he is being appreciated and cherished, when he knows that parents and teachers love him and have his well-being at heart, then the child in turn will be willing to accept the unavoidable limits which have to be set at times.

As a guideline for truthfulness and kindness, I would like to quote the following:

> *"Everything we say has to be true,*
> *Yet not everything which is true can be said."*

Out of consideration for the other person, we should at times keep our silence.

More than anything else, in order for the truth to be accepted, there has to be great trust.

g. The children who miss school because they are sick so much (Case# 264, p.141).

4. Further Consequences

1. Repeating a grade (Case# 1430, p.138.

2. Transfer from college preparatory courses to a less academic curriculum (Case#153, p.138).

My observations show that more than half of the students who are taking the easy courses in high school are not lacking in intelligence, but in health and well-being, or are forced to do so because of problems in their home environment.

In both cases I have come to the conclusion that the real reason is the damage done by the zones of disturbance to the children, and in some cases to the parents.

Needless to say, other factors can be responsible.

I only want to mention the lack of sleep and the fidgetiness caused by daily television viewing, especially in the evening.

3. Transfer into the educationally handicapped programme.

Brain damaged people - and also epileptics - react particularly strongly to zones of disturbance.

A healthful place to sleep and work is particularly important for them during their school years and also later on in life, so that they can make optimal use of the opportunities offered them, and also to forestall convulsions.

I have observed 15 people with epileptic seizures, or with seizures similar to epilepsy, and in every case I found the presence of a zone of disturbance at the site of the bed or at the place of work.

4. The place for homework was also situated above a disturbed area in some cases (Case# 327, p.145).

I saw some children who were not able to remain at that place for any length of time, and who would give any excuse - including that there was no more homework - to be able to leave.

An absolutely undisturbed, quiet place to do homework is imperative for successful studying.

5. The location of the desk in school (No. 519, p.145) is also of importance.

This can become very important because students may have to sit for quite a long time, in some cases even for a year, on the same spot. That spot may be located above a zone of disturbance.

I saw children who sat apathetically at their desk for a whole year (Case# 1247, p.146), who looked 'out of it', and who even fainted in two cases (Case# 519, p.145).

Every time we have found that they sat above a crossing. Such places also caused weeping 'without a reason', stomach aches and vomiting.

In a particularly difficult case, I could see that the child came to hate school so much that he refused to go. The parents used gentle persuasion, coercion, all to no avail.

Only after the child was relocated to a good place at home and in school did everything change for the better for him.

6. Bed wetting (Case# 120, p.147). Many factors come together in bed wetting, including psychological ones.

However, I found that in the 53 cases which I studied, a zone of disturbance was always present.

After that factor was removed, a rapid improvement could be seen, and in some cases even an immediate cure. One mother wrote to me, *"My expectations were surpassed by far"*.

7. Differences in siblings (Case# 542, p.147). *"Take your brother (or sister) as an example".* This is told to some children again and again, by parents and teachers.

My observation has been that those children who are less successful than their siblings are often the victims of damaging influences from the earth, and simply did not have the energy it takes to succeed.

8. Good performance in school, despite the disturbed fields ?

Yes, it happens ! I noticed that some students did not suffer intellectually, but did well in school, occasionally even very well. However, they did not feel well physically.

I wonder whether those students might not have done even more outstanding work if their energy had not been drained so much.

They certainly could have achieved the same level without so much effort, and in less time.

They would have had more free time to play outside, for sports, for daydreaming and leisure, for some artistic activities, for human contacts, and for being friendly and helpful.

We see it in the working world as well as in school that people are capable of outstanding achievements, even though their family life is stressful or they suffer from their difficulties.

A robust disposition or a good mental attitude can bridge those situations.

But the price is effort, waste of energy, and the inability to work to one's full potential in all areas of life.

Why pay such a high price, when help is possible ?

And with zones of disturbance, help is so easily attained !

9. <u>Again and again we hear the complaint that students are 'made to work too hard'.</u>

Often the teacher is blamed.

But the real reason is often that the student has been weakened physically and mentally by zones of disturbance he has been exposed to, so that he is not capable of doing justice to the things daily life demands of him.

When he is tired, he looks out of the window, when he wastes his time, when he has to go over and over material before he can remember it, then he will not be able to do his work in the allotted time.

But when he feels well and is in good spirits, then he can usually work faster and is able to cope with daily life.

10. <u>Reproach.</u> Since I have put so much emphasis on the influence of the zones of disturbance as the real reason for the failure of so many students in different areas, I have been reproached for being too lenient with students and too protective, and for not valuing their education enough in regard to strength of character, self-sufficiency, attainment of physical fitness, moderation and restraint.

On the contrary, I set high value on those aspects of education and have stressed them in my contacts with students during my 30 years as a teacher.

But I am of the opinion that some of the children suffer from unjust disapproval, threats and punishment.

In some of these instances it would be helpful to look for the real reason for the difficulties and the failures, so that the discomfort of the children could be alleviated.

I myself am convinced that education can be successful only if there is a good foundation of restful and sufficient sleep, and physical and emotional well-being.

Children need to be able to do what is good and necessary for them in a happy and cooperative frame of mind.

Many a 'troublemaker', many children who are aggressive, moody and just plain difficult, become even-tempered, harmonious, generally pleasant people to be with once they are removed from exposure to zones of disturbance.

11. It is sometimes said that 'model students' will not be able to cope with life later on, whereas bad students will turn out to be capable adults.

That is an over-generalization which is actually not correct.

Most 'model students' are not only conscientious students but are also successful in their interaction with their peers.

And later on in life they tend to perform well and hold responsible positions.

However, there is a grain of truth in this statement, and it is borne out in some cases.

First of all, there is the possibility that children and parents, and children and teachers, have a difficult time together personally.

Second, we all know that some people enjoy practical work more than theoretical learning.

And third, and this third factor I have observed over and over again, we find that children, as soon as they finish school, will move away.

We now deal with an alteration of the zones of disturbance - to the disadvantage of some, to the advantage of others.

Thus, we can better understand why a happy, capable and successful student might have a difficult time running his life later on and why a 'problem child' might in the end do very well.

12. I draw similar conclusions in regard to high school and university students as to students in the lower grades.

13. What results occurred after the bed or desk was moved ?
    a. Sleep habits improved at once in almost all the children's cases.
    b. Appetite improved, especially for breakfast.
    c. Better general health and well-being.
    d. Attention span and interest in learning improved at once, especially in those subjects where the pupil was not too far behind.
    e. Improved capacity for thinking and remembering.
    f. In cases where the damage from zones of disturbance had lasted for only a short time, like a few months or one year at the most, the students' performance in school improved immediately.
    g. Gradually improved performance in almost all the other areas of study also.

Students who have been disadvantaged because of zones of disturbance in the important early years will, of course, have considerable gaps in their knowledge, and in general have a hard time working up to grade level.

They will have to work quite hard and it will take some time before their scholastic performance becomes satisfactory.

14. Percentage. In 95% of the cases which I have examined and which involved failure in school, I found the presence of zones of disturbance to be a contributing factor.

15. What assistance can a teacher give, even though he himself might not be able to do any dowsing ?

(a). He can institute the concept of the 'rotating classroom', by asking students to change seats every three to four weeks.

In this way, we can be sure that no student will be exposed for the duration of the school year to a geopathic crossing.

Needless to say, some of the 'radiated places' within the classroom will have to be occupied.

However, in cases where an examination is conducted, it is definitely possible to arrange the desks in such a way that no student will have to sit above a strong crossing.

(b). Every teacher is eager to facilitate the learning process in his students. Therefore it is important that he finds the time to inquire about the physical and mental state of health of his students from time to time. The time it takes him to do this is well spent.

For what use is the urging, the coaxing, and the blaming, if indeed the student is incapable of learning and of retaining what he has learned, because of circumstances from the outside ?

I have posed ten questions, based on the ten indicators for the presence of pathogenic zones, to the children of the first four grades of the intermediate school (see page 74).

Those children were 10 years old. I jotted down the name of every student who responded to the different questions. (I have kept the list of names and the notes I made in shorthand).

(c). Advice for moving the bed 'for better or worse' or for 'just in case'.

I gave the children a few examples and said, *"I believe that those who raised their hands owe their discomforts and complaints to the zones of disturbance. Please, talk to your parents about it. If your house is built on a slope, I want you to put the bed sideways to the slope, not pointed downwards, because of the 'pushing effect' of the water currents. And sometimes it is even enough to move the bed as little as half a metre or one metre".*

(d). Finding out about the results. After three weeks, I talked again to all the children whose names I had taken down.

Most of them had obtained permission from their parents to move the bed around, and most of them reported that they felt better, and that they ate more with more pleasure.

Such a splendid success came as a total surprise!

Kurt said, *"Now I just lie down and fall asleep right away"*.

And Kurt was a child who had experienced difficulty falling asleep for the past four years, and who consequently was nervous and in ill health and who had many failures at home and in school.

Maria, who had vomited every morning for years, said *"Since the bed has been moved I have not thrown up even once"*.

Michaela brought me a letter her parents had written: *"... her state of health has improved considerably"*.

Richard's parents sent me a letter in which they stressed the 'quiet sleep' of their son.

(e). In total, 120 children were asked how they felt, and 52 of them (43%) showed definite symptoms of zones of disturbance.

Of those, 48 pupils experienced remarkable improvement in their well-being after the bed was moved in the haphazard way I described above !

But one pupil said the following: *"before the bed was moved I always had a headache when I woke up. Now I have a stomach ache."*

I told her that she was probably lying above a crossing in the middle of her bed, and I encouraged her to ask her parents to move the bed still further.

And in case this was not successful, then her parents could ask me to check their house and find the place best suited for her.

Teachers who cannot do these examinations can always recommend a good dowser.

(f). Talking to the parents. There are situations where I consider it important to talk directly to the parents; for example in the case of particularly sensitive children, or children under very difficult circumstances; in cases where a student fails suddenly and does not improve again, despite my recommendation to move the bed; and in cases where the parents don't see the purpose of the procedure and thus do not allow the child to move the bed.

In all of these instances I request an interview with the parents in the hope that this might bring about the desired result.

I am stressing this whole subject so that teachers and parents can become aware of its seriousness and importance and thus might earnestly consider what steps should be taken to help the child.

(g). Prudent foresight is imperative in dealing with children.

We should not talk about it too often, so as to trigger a 'radiation neurosis' in the child.

Also, the children must not get the idea that they can use this as an excuse at every opportunity.

On the contrary, we need to calm them and keep their attention off these problems, perhaps pointing out to them that there is also something like a spiritual radiation which emanates from certain people.

In the presence of such people everyone feels peaceful and uplifted at the same time, and they should strive towards becoming people like that themselves.

Years ago, I talked to my students once briefly about the influence of the zones of disturbance. I asked about their sleep patterns and made notes of what they answered.

Everything else I pursued during my time off at weekends and during vacations.

I made contact with the parents of those students who seemed to suffer most from the disturbances. The parents then asked me for a specific examination of their living quarters.

The above-mentioned extensive investigation of children in four grades was done rather recently, with a view to the present scientific presentation.

Because of a lack of time and energy, I was unable to help personally in every case. Thus, it occurred to me to recommend moving the bed 'for better or worse'.

The 'rotating classroom' is being continued by many teachers once a month, without giving any particular reason for it.

This procedure is also justified in view of the different lighting conditions in a classroom.

And those children who would like to sit together again can easily be moved together.

Some teachers have been willing to follow the suggestions I made several years ago in personal discussions with them and in public lectures.

I know for sure that some other teachers (dowsers - five of whom I know personally) have also made the same observations in their classrooms. They too achieved valuable results.

But so far I do not know of anything that has been published about these results.

5. Teachers, University Professors and School
Principals Exposed to Zones of Disturbance
(13 case histories from Part III)

1. The Teacher (Case# 1299, p.149)

The state of health of the teacher has, of course, a great influence on the performance of his students.

It makes a difference whether a teacher is happy, relaxed, enjoying his work and patient, or whether he is depressed, nervous, tired and short of concentration due to the detrimental effects of zones of disturbance.

Because of his ill health he may stay home sick and the children will have to deal with substitute teachers for much of the time.

As long as the teacher has a place to sleep which is free of interferences, then he need not be concerned about the zones of disturbance in the classroom, since he changes his position all the time while teaching.

2. High School Teacher and University Professor

(Case# 1380, p.111) These tend to occupy the same place for much longer periods of time, during lectures and also during exams.

For their benefit, as well as for the well-being of the students, it is important for these locations to be free of radiation.

A teacher, overly sensitive or even ill, and a student who is not feeling up to par and who is therefore nervous, distracted and ill at ease, can be responsible in more than one case for low test scores.

It is important for teachers and students to avoid pathogenic locations, especially during periods of stress.

3. The location of the teacher's desk needs to be investigated.

The teacher tends to spend hours in the afternoon correcting papers and preparing lessons.

The energy drain due to a pathogenic location needs to be avoided.

4. It is imperative that the principal or headmaster occupy an office free of radiation.

I have had the opportunity to examine several offices where one principal after the other became ill and was forced into premature retirement.   In each case a zone of disturbance was present.

A principal who is feeling energetic and able to work hard without undue fatigue will create an atmosphere in the school where students and teachers will be eager to work together.

Several principals assured me that they began to feel much better right after the desk was moved to another part of the office.

6. Plans for the Future

1. It is important that school districts, teachers, colleagues and other teacher-training institutions become cognizant of zones of disturbance through workshops, conferences and lectures with slide presentations.

Parents need to be informed during PTA meetings, again with lectures and case presentations, and the children need to have the phenomenon explained to them.

2. <u>Some sensitive teachers need to be trained</u> in the use of the dowsing rod.

One school district had already arranged for me to give my lecture 'Zones of Disturbance in Schools' to about 40 participants in a workshop for teachers, and to augment it with slides.

A lively and stimulating discussion followed. A short documentary film was made of the workshop.

My colleague Helmut Boehm knew how to give the film the necessary psychological emphasis and also how to handle the subject factually and objectively.

My task was to ask the 'ten questions' I have enumerated earlier for use in the classroom.

Also, I was to examine the bedroom of two of the children who responded in the affirmative most often to these questions.

Indeed, the bed of Christine 0. stood directly above a Curry crossing.

Her mother told me:

"There was always that question nagging at me; why does that child have no appetite in the morning, and why is she always so nervous ?"

Gottfried E's bed actually stood over a double crossing (water current crossing and Curry crossing).

No wonder the child was so ill-tempered, did not make friends, was sick a lot, did so poorly in school that he had to stay after class for many an afternoon, and had very poor sleeping habits.

Each child was allowed to move his bed to another place, free from damaging rays.

Three weeks later I learned how much better everything was going for them.

I am hopeful that my empirical investigations have uncovered the real reason for so many school failures, and they will contribute in at least a small way to the well-being of young people and to the progress of science.

7. Building of Schools and School Furniture

The leading German environmentalist, Dr. Werner Kauffman, recommended the inclusion in the new edition of my book of some of the suggestions in regard to the importance of building materials and furniture used in schools.

I would like to take this opportunity to thank him for his contributions and also for the information he has allowed me to use. The following pages were written by Dr. Kauffman.

Geobiology, Construction Biology,
Environmentology and School Architecture

'Tu felix Austria'...that's what comes to mind every time I put down Käthe Bachler's book.

That's the country with so much intellectual freedom that even 50 years ago Prof. Bier from Berlin and Dr. Schreiber, a dowser from the public health department, went to the oldest German university together, to the University of Prague, along with Professor Fuerth of Prague, to explore in depth the physical influences involved in the turning of the dowsing rod.

And that's the country where the phenomenon of the electric charge of living cells could be explored, where men like Keller, Gickelhorn and Pischinger could pursue their biophysical work with all the freedom necessary for objective investigation.

Later, their work was continued with the same thoroughness at the University of Vienna.

I am in a position to confirm every word and every observation made by Käthe Bachler.

We (my friends and I) are so gratified with the reports of her research - from corneitis to the disintegration of the family, from the small child fleeing the radiated places to the wife who runs away from home in a state of panic.

In writing this book, Käthe Bachler shows much personal perseverance and devotion and the expenditure of so much personal energy that it can easily lead to a state of exhaustion, as Ms. Bachler has described from her personal experience.

This work does not deal with hypotheses, but produces proofs, and they have to be given attention when it comes to the design and construction of facilities which house computers and similar electronic equipment.

In some places (Denmark and Cologne), the electrical charge (ions) in the classroom was tested and correlated with the productivity of the students and with their propensity to illness.

The Swedish Academy of Science has examined several hundred apartments and houses in regard to ion levels in the air in relation to the kind of materials used in the building.

Summarized in one sentence, the results were, *"The greater the atomic density of the building material, the stronger the electric charge of the air in that building."*

Air which is overloaded with charge causes fatigue and lack of concentration. That happens when the classrooms are furnished with too many synthetic materials, from the carpets to the plastic tables and seats.

The Max-Planck Institute for Work Physiology (Dortmund/ Germany) showed that female workers sitting at tables covered with plastic materials eventually suffer from circulatory problems in their arms.

Observant parents have noticed that their children showed signs of fatigue more quickly when the shabby looking wooden table top was replaced with a nice looking formica top.

That trend was quickly reversed when a solid old wooden board was reintroduced.

But why put all this information into a book ?

We have found schools located next to huge power stations and learned that some children were fainting during school hours.

We have seen schools which were built like greenhouses - cement, steel, large amounts of glass and artificial materials.

Earth Radiation

116

Children and teachers suffered from this 'greenhouse effect' and it took much ingenuity to prevent the sun from overheating the rooms.

In 1970, there was an international congress for 'Building Biology' organized by the Institute for Building Research in Vienna. In Germany there have been several symposia for architectural medicine.

Again and again we hear the complaint from architects that while they are building thousands of houses and buildings, they are being criticized repeatedly.

They complain that nobody seems able to tell them beforehand how they should build. This book is not the place to give even a short version of a 'building biology for schools'. Yet schools are being built for the use of several generations. Unfortunately, stress and its consequences on the performance of each generation begins in the classroom.

Therefore, I want to take this opportunity to emphasize that apart from the geobiological circumstances - which have been discussed in detail in this book - some of their factors need to be dealt with, since they influence the environment of the classroom a great deal.

Naturally, neither teachers nor physicians can be expected to examine the sleeping areas of their students or patients.

But the generation growing up now, which has to live all the time with the impact of those environmental influences, has a right to find out about the knowledge and research in regard to these phenomena. As an introduction I want to quote a few definitions.

In the 'Encyclopaedia of Physics' by Hermann Franke, D.T.V., we find under 'earth rays': *radiation which emanates from the earth because of the presence of radioactive substances*.

We have conducted measurements with special instruments and could show that 'thermal neutron rays' also emanate from the locations of disturbance.

Thermal neutron rays were also the cause of cancer after the atomic bombs were dropped on Japan.

We know from American measurements which were taken in the area around Neuss and Xanten that every historical movement of the earth (Roman camps, buildings, graves and buried weapons) can be measured from the surface of the earth with a proton resonance magnometer.

Likewise, every subterranean water current, even if it is only of molecular scale (1 metre in 24 hours) can be measured and has a biological effect.

The Austrian Institute for Building Research reports in the book 'Dampness of Buildings' that movements of water within the earth produce friction which in turn produces electricity.

This electricity goes up with the walls and pulls water molecules along. We get the phenomenon of 'building dampness' (electro-osmosis), which can be measured as an electric force of approximately one volt.

Above water currents in the earth we see the presence of ionic walls, in some cases as high as several thousand metres according to Dr. Buerklin, Director of the electrical power station in Bamberg, Germany (this information was given to me personally).

All those circumstances influence the ion levels of the living space and thus are biologically important.

They produce, through nuclear magnetic resonance (acting on the protons in the water), changes in the pH of the lymphatic fluid of the body.

In 'Newest Results on Terrestrial Rays Outside and in the Home', a chart published by the Ministry of the Interior in 1977, we learn for the first time how much the intensity of the rays increases in our homes because of the 'inhibiting capacity' of the building material.

According to the Swedish Academy of Science, there exists a several hundredfold difference between a wooden house and one built from concrete, as far as the ionization of the air retained in the rooms.

Outside we have air which carries opposite charges, and the oxygen of the air is continually activated by ultraviolet rays from the sun.

Inside the rooms of a building, these relationships change considerably; the air is influenced to some extent by static charge from surfaces made of artificial materials.

Juxtaposing a wall made of glass and one made of synthetic material can create a potential difference as great as 6,000 volts.

People exposed to such voltages experience marked discomfort and can undergo considerable changes (Dr. Josef Eichmaier, Institute of Technology, Munich).

This may also shed some light on the fact that many children nowadays, living in nurseries with a predominance of 'easy to take care of' materials, become nervous and lack curiosity and exuberance.

Radio, TV, loudspeakers (magnets), and electrical and battery-operated alarm clocks should not be near the bed, especially not near the head, since they upset the hormonal balance. Their distance ought to be at least two metres, and their influence even penetrates a wall.

We do not favour the kinds of rooms so much in vogue with young people, which are decorated almost entirely with artificial fibres.

Nor do we favour tables made of plastic, chairs made with plastic materials, or swivel chairs with steel screws which will become magnetic.

We have met several mayors of cities who, without our prodding, ordered the removal of artificial material after they became aware of how just much the intellectual capacity of the students had diminished in modern school houses.

They returned to good old hardwood floors, without even plastic sealers.

Beginning with each meadow (as part of the examination of the planned building site) and ending with the finished building, we have examined villages, hospitals, clinics, and apartment complexes where children grow up, and we have served as biological and ecological consultants.

We are very aware of the mistakes of modern architecture.

Ms. Käthe Bachler selected a truly controversial subject for herself. But we are convinced that the truth will eventually be heard:

"Walls and windows and doors make up a house, but the space inside makes its true nature."

Dr. Werner Kaufmann Altzbach, 1978.

I hope that Dr. Kaufmann's valuable contribution will be met with interest and understanding.

May those who are in a position of responsibility, mayors, school principals and architects, pay more attention to this subject while the buildings are still in the initial planning stages.

I also want to point out that Dr. Kaufman has given an excellent lecture 'The Microclimate and its Significance for the Health of Children' (published by Dr. Kaufman, Atzbach).

The Right Size of School Furniture

In this connection I would like to address myself to a problem which has been brought home to me again and again in my capacity as a teacher for so many years. I have always felt sorry for the students who had to suffer because of it.

Most classrooms are furnished with standard size desks, chairs and tables. Thus, some short students have to sit in school all day with their feet dangling in the air because the seat is too high for them.

While writing, they have to pull up their arms and shoulders since the writing surface is too high for them. Most adults simply would not able to tolerate this.

And in the same classroom we find some tall students who have to sit crooked and lopsided in the desks and chairs because they cannot find a comfortable place for their long legs.

They run the risk of damaging their spines permanently; and furthermore, they have to write for hours stooped over since the writing surface is too low for them.

The furniture was designed for an average-sized child.

Nobody took into account the fact that every class has children taller and shorter than the average.

Every physician and school psychologist knows that for optimal health, for feeling well, for normal development and for a high performance level, the size of the furniture has to match the size of the students.

Thus every classroom should have some smaller furniture in front and some larger furniture in the back. It is more important to have the correct size than the same size.

I very much hope that more attention will be paid to this important subject as time goes on. There are already some pertinent sources of information on the market to serve as guidelines.

Part III - CASE HISTORIES AND STATISTICAL INFORMATION

Introduction

I will limit myself to just a few examples out of the wealth of case histories I have accumulated.

Otherwise, the book would become too voluminous and too expensive.

I could easily add many similar examples to every factual account presented here.

I am aware that people have very little time for reading nowadays.

Therefore, my aim has been to keep the book as brief as possible.

However, the amount of material I have included in this part of the book seemed absolutely essential, in order to provide proof for the contributory role of terrestrial influences to many cases of illness.

The factual material is ordered in the following way: first, reactions of animals; then reactions of humans in general.

After that, the examples which belong to the section 'school failures', followed by examples of different organ diseases, ordered into appropriate groups.

Each one of these groups contains a statistical breakdown and a summary.

At the end I have added examples of pathology, caused by pathogenic seating arrangements or by pathogenic locations in which people have to stand for a long time.

The statements which accompany the drawings are highly simplified, often incomplete, or just mere indications.

As I said before, I chose to write down exactly what people told me. Some of it they did not tell me, of course.

Nevertheless, I believe the observations to be important enough to be included in detail in this book.

Case# 1553c. Dogs seek a 'good' place.

Christian, a very sensitive young man, changed his room (I). Soon he became tired, complained of headaches, and lost his appetite.

After three months, he came down with severe influenza, followed by meningitis. He could not stand being in bed, and just walked around in his room.

He was hospitalized for three weeks. There he was able to sleep, and in general felt better, and the pains subsided.

As soon as he was home again, the headaches reappeared and he felt the same exhaustion as before.

Two weeks later I was asked by his parents to examine the place where he slept. An intersection of zones of disturbance lay directly under his head !

The bed was moved immediately into the other corner of the room which was free of 'radiation'.

The skeptical young man performed a test. He fetched his big dog, lured him into the 'radiated' corner where previously the bed had stood, put a warm blanket on the floor, and gave the command to the dog to lie down there and to stay. Then he left the room.

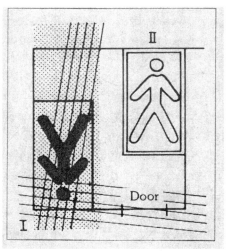

When he returned five minutes later he found the dog lying on his bed on the place free of radiation (II).

The critical young man laughed when he told us of his experiment to use his dog as the control for my statements.

Christian slept well from then on, the headaches went, and he soon regained his previous state of health.

Case# 663.   The cat is a 'radiation seeker'

She loves intersections of zones of disturbance the most !

She always seeks out beds which stand above crossings of zones of disturbance. See the following illustrations:

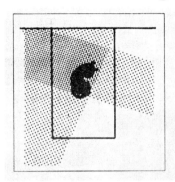
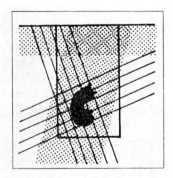

Irene, 9 years old, suffered from chronic headaches and abdominal pains.
After the bed was moved, recovery followed quickly.

Mr. A. suffered from constant backaches.
A man whose bedroom was located exactly above Mr. A.'s bedroom died of cancer.

Case# 1293b. Fish will react.

The aquarium stood at the same spot for 18 months. The small tropical fish always crowded into the left corner of the aquarium. Furthermore, they ate their eggs.

Previously the aquarium had been located in a different room, free of radiation.
There they swam all around in their aquarium and spawned three times, producing healthy young fish.

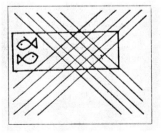

The aquarium was finally relocated back to the old position.

A letter of December 16th, 1973 says:

"Since we moved the aquarium back into the old room, the fish enjoy swimming throughout the length and breadth of their tank, laid eggs after four weeks, and took good care of their young. Dr. G. R., Biologieprofessor."

My examination of 3,000 residences yielded the following observations:

1. Influences from the earth and their effects fall into the following categories, ranked according to increasing intensity (strength of effect):

C (= Curry bands/grid)
Nervousness, mild insomnia and spasms or convulsions possible.

W (= water vein/current)
Feeling cold and tired, rheumatism possible.

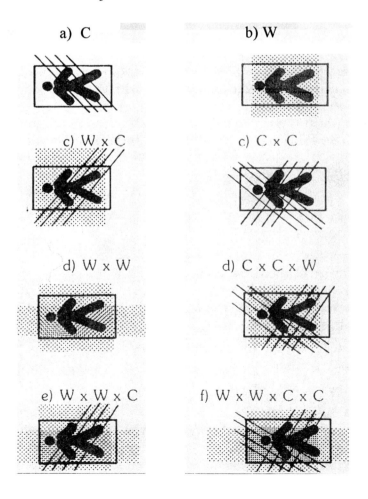

a) C

b) W

c) W x C

c) C x C

d) W x W

d) C x C x W

e) W x W x C

f) W x W x C x C

In the range of b to f, we expect severe sleep disturbances, spasms and serious illnesses.

2. Influences from the earth and their effects, ranked according to their decreasing <u>frequency</u> of occurrence as pathogenic factors:

a.   C x C x W
b.   W x C
c.   C x C
d.   W
e.   C
f.   W x W
g.   W x W x C
h.   W x W x W x C x C

    (combination h. was observed in only 0.8% of the cases).

I used the compass in all of my examinations of residences. In every case I noticed that the curry strips were aligned between the points of the compass, that is, NE-SW, NW-SE.

I marked them in my sketches in the same way. However, I thought it would be unnecessary to indicate the points of the compass in every drawing.

It should be understood that if a house is aligned 'in between' the compass directions, the Curry strips would then run parallel to the walls.

1. Firsthand Records Concerning Babies and Young Children

<u>Case# 610. Premature birth</u>

Gall bladder, cramps and pain in the feet, premature delivery.

The doctor believed that without the appropriate measures, the foetus would have been aborted.

The dowser said: *"The child wanted to flee already from the uterus."*

The child was born after 6½ months of pregnancy.

The child cried most of the time, had convulsions, was restless.

The mother had to get up at night as often as 20 times to quiet the baby.

After the bed was moved to another place, there was improvement.

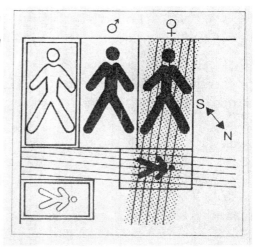

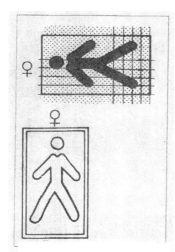

Case# 1249. The much-hoped-for child was finally born !

Mrs. N. waited in vain for a child over a period of 12 years.

She suffered a tubal pregnancy and suffered from abdominal problems. The physician recommended an examination of the house.

A new location for the bed was recommended, and the woman recovered.

Five months later she became pregnant; the pregnancy and delivery were uneventful.

The baby was put in a place free from radiation and she progressed very well. Mathilde is now a year old (in 1977) and is a happy, bouncing baby.

Case# 102. Dorli died from convulsions.

Little Dorli was only a few months old. During pregnancy, her mother had slept over a zone of disturbance crossing.

Thus, Dorli was a small and frail infant. The mother became ill and had to be hospitalized. The child was put into a foster home.

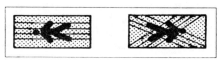

Home   **Foster Home**

Dorli became very ill in the first foster home and was taken to another one. There her condition became worse, and she developed convulsions. She died two months later.

Case# 180. Twin, 14 months old, flees from his bed.

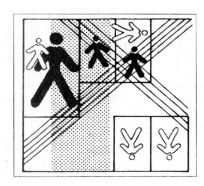

George could not sleep, and he cried until his mother put him next to her.   Dieter fled his Curry crossing and then he slept well !

His mother suffered from insomnia and also from a kidney ailment. His father had previously slept above the Curry crossing, and during that time he was very nervous.

After relocating the bed, the twin slept peacefully in the middle of his crib.

Case# 660. The ten-month-old baby was tied to his crib.

The parents were afraid he might fall out of bed, because he stood up again and again.

When in his playpen, he only occupied the half which was 'free of radiation', never the half above the Curry strip.

The father finally phoned me: *"Since we moved the bed, we have had no problem with his sleeping and he is healthy and robust."*

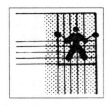

Case# 542. Two-year-old.

He avoided the zones of disturbance in his sleep
and put his head on the north side of the bed. The
concerned grandfather, unfortunately, turned their
child around several times every night.

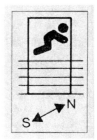

When the bed was moved, the sleep was
undisturbed.

If at all possible, the head should point north
(children as well as adults).

Case# 192. A happy Austrian family.

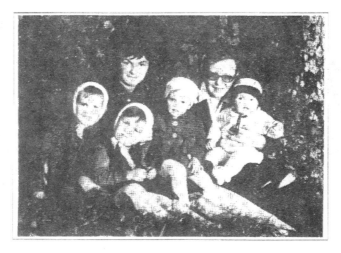

Only little Heartha (second child from right) cried every night,
and she was sick a great deal.

Her eyes show the fear with which she looks
out into the world.

Her bed stood above a zone of disturbance
and a crossing !

[*Apologies for the quality of the photographs.*
The originals were not available for this edition.]

After a year I received a letter with a photograph. Heartha (the first child on the right) was thriving in her new sleeping place.

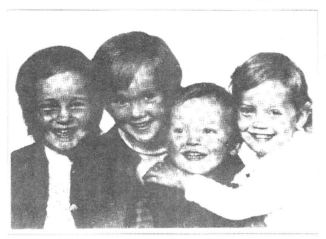

Case# 1523. Martin was fortunate after his birth !

Both parents have been sleeping 'here', and both suffer from different ailments.

The mother had three miscarriages.

Only with much medical help and many precautions did she succeed in carrying the next child to term.

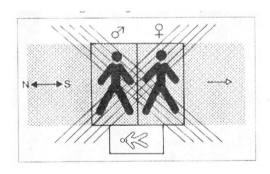

Martin was weak at birth, and suffered from gastrointestinal problems. He vomited a great deal.

However, by sheer coincidence, he was put in a place free of radiation.

Thus he was able to gain weight and strength, and after two months he was a happy and healthy baby.

He is now 18 months old.

Case# 1370b. Michaela, 18 months old,

took on a squatting or kneeling
position much of the time, and would
rock back and forth.

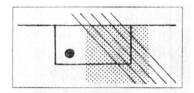

Case# 295. Elfi, 2 years old,

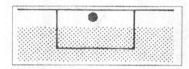

appeared to want to climb up the wall,
especially during full moon

Case# 1457. Two children in Tyrol.

Klemens, two years old, slept fitfully,
suffered from coughing and frequently threw
up during the night, never during the day.

Verena did well for two months, but then
was lying above water for six weeks. She
slept poorly, had little appetite, and vomited
frequently.

New locations for the beds resulted in both
children sleeping well, no more vomiting,
and their development was normal (from
their father's letter).

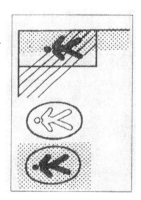

Case# 1177. Change of location of bed for 'good measure'.

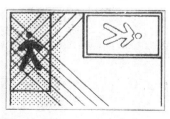

This helped little Manfred immediately
with his severe asthma and his
suffocating attacks.

Case# 732. 'Crying without any apparent reason'.

A five year old girl woke up crying every morning; during the day she was often moody and 'hard to take'.

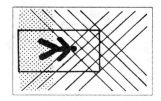

She often hit herself on the head, and whenever she did this she would faint.

After the bed was moved, she recovered completely within a short time.

 Case# 159. 4 yr old boy refused to sit at the table during meals.

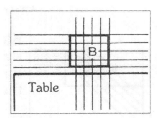

His parents were annoyed with him.

Once the table was moved to another corner of the room, he remained at the table.

A two-year-old girl slept fitfully during the night.

Her father, a municipal judge in Salzburg, wrote to me: *"On your advice we moved our little daughter's bed just 30 cms.*

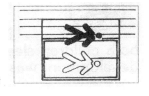

The following night she was able to sleep quietly and uninterruptedly for the first time in a long, long time.

This demonstration conquered my initial skepticism about your theory."

Case# 403. Stuttering.

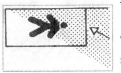

This child was late to walk and talk, and he stuttered until, at the age of six, he was moved to a better sleeping place.

2. Firsthand Accounts Concerning School-age Children

Case# 201. The school psychologist was puzzled.

During the first and second year of the child's life, his development seemed retarded, and he did not talk at all.

During the third to sixth year of life, the child was mentally retarded.

The school psychologist's judgement was *"This child needs to be put into a school for the handicapped."*

Through sheer coincidence, the child's bed was moved.

Suddenly all the effort and care of his intelligent mother brought measurable success.

The child progressed in all areas of his life.

He was put into a regular grammar school on a trial basis. To everyone's surprise, he came home with 'Good' on his first report card.

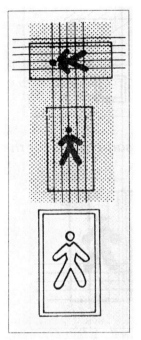

Case# 1507a. A first grader at School.

Ingeborg slept well and ate a good breakfast.

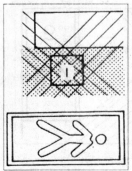

Four months after she started school, she began to look pale and had no appetite for lunch.

She was tired in school, restless and grouchy.

She said, *"I don't like anything anymore."*

Though obviously intelligent, her performance in school was poor.

After she was assigned to another desk, she said, *"I had a nice time today."*

Case#1507b. Ingebord had two places for doing homework.

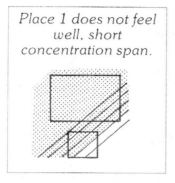

Place 1 does not feel well. short concentration span.

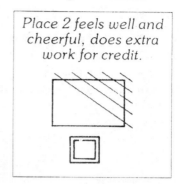

Place 2 feels well and cheerful, does extra work for credit.

Case# 984. He has slept in the same place for 2 years.

Since then Rudi, 10 years old, has complained about being cold in bed and stomach aches.

He is anxious, sick a lot and his school attendance is poor.

Soon after his bed was moved, there was a marked improvement in all areas.

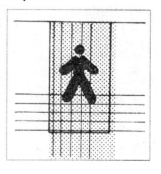

Case# 236. Monica, 10 yrs old, suffers from nausea and vomiting.

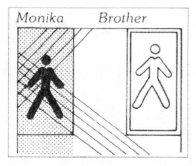

Monika   Brother

She had to leave the classroom frequently.

I asked whether she had medical attention.

Her reply was, *"Yes, but the doctor said that nothing worked with me, that he had tried everything, that I had a nervous stomach and nothing could be done about it".*

Monica failed in school also.   I visited her parents, who asked me to investigate the place where Monica slept.

Her bed, indeed, stood above a Curry crossing and a water current.

Her brother enjoyed a good place to sleep and was healthy.

My recommendation was to put Monica in a bunk bed above her brother's.

The next morning Monica announced that she had slept well and felt better.

Soon her health recovered and she became successful in school.

Case# 1156. Jane's parents resented every teacher.

They were convinced that it was the fault of the teacher that their daughter woke up trembling every morning.

Jane ran a fever frequently in the morning, vomited, could not eat, was always tired, had circulatory problems and missed a lot of school.

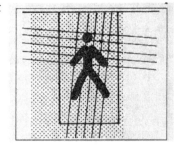

She was far behind in her studies and therefore often discouraged and unhappy.

Her teacher asked her to have the bed examined.

After the bed was moved, she recovered rapidly.

Case# 101. Irmtraud slept above 'pushing water'.

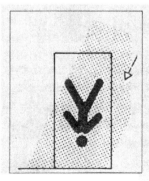

This resulted in nightmares, running out of her room, depression and lack of appetite.

Her mother, a pharmacist, wrote: *"The child used to come into my room one or two times every night, anxious because of nightmares.*

Often she woke up crying in the morning.

Now she sleeps peacefully, the blankets stay on, and she wakes up alert and refreshed.

Since we have moved her bed she feels much better.

The first reaction was that she was positively hungry... We cannot thank you enough !"

Case# 632. Maria was given to sleepwalking.

Maria, 12 years old, was very small, very pale, and sick much of the time, suffering from severe stomach pains.

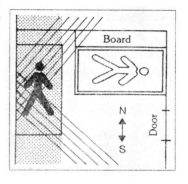

She had a strong dislike for her bed, was reluctant to go to bed at night, and was unable to go to sleep for hours much of the time.

She missed school frequently and was far behind, and had a hard time learning. The bed was relocated. Her mother wrote three months later:

"Maria looks so much better and in general so different, and she actually feels better and does not mind going to bed ... her schoolwork, too, has much improved".

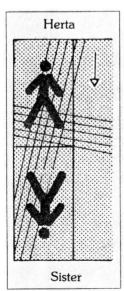

Case# 658. Herta is very nervous

She is 13 years old and shakes with fear.

She is small, frail, cries easily and her school attendance is irregular.

She never falls asleep before 11 pm.

She is easily frustrated and reluctant to try anything new.

Result of the examination: three-metre wide pulling water current and Curry crossing.

Herta's sister too is delicate and sick a great deal. Both girls were moved into another room.

The sleeping pattern changed for the better immediately, they became stronger physically, and their well-being improved rapidly.

Case# 1259b. "Nerve pills" were needed for the 10 year-old !

Reinhard, 10 years old, suffered from severe headaches, disturbed sleep, marked nervousness and tiredness.

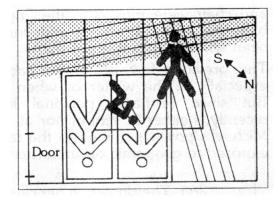

His bed was moved, and he slept better immediately and in general felt better and looked healthier.

Gerlinde, 6 years old, avoided the problem !

She turned around in her bed during sleep and moved to a different spot. She stayed well.

Case# 1741. Michael, 13, has attacks of migraine.

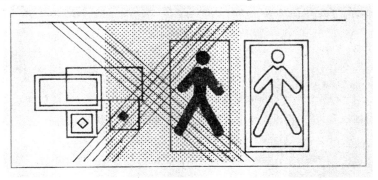

His father, a school principal, wrote on December 3, 1975: *"The most convincing and positive change occurred with our son Michael.*

Ever since his bed, desk, and chair were moved to the 'right' place, he has not had one single attack of migraine.

In fact, he has not been sick in any way since then.

The previous few years, he had suffered from colds, especially in the winter or when the weather changed.

But since Michael's personal life has not changed recently, neither in school nor at home, I have to credit Michael's positive change to the fact that he is no longer exposed to geopathic disturbances".

Case# 265. The slowest in her class, 10 years old.

In my capacity as a teacher, I experienced the following:

We had to wait for her forever, before we could clean the blackboard. I asked her how she slept.

She told me: *"I fall asleep very late. And often I fall out of bed with all of my blankets and then I continue to sleep on the floor".*

The parents reported: *"Our child is an 'rh-factor child' and has been anaemic from birth".*

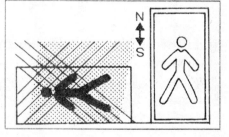

Yes, that was definitely one factor of her difficulty; the second cause was the crossing of two zones of disturbance.

The bed was changed. Restful sleep at once, feeling better in general, hungry at mealtimes !

Soon her tempo at work improved, and so did her grades.

Five months later she had rosy cheeks and was a picture of health.

Case# 772.   Pupil K, 14, does no homework.

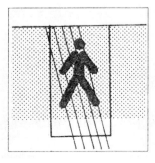

At home she sits listlessly at the table, stares into space, does not get anything done.

She fails in school, despite her intelligence.

She has great trouble falling asleep.

She misses many schooldays.

The bed was put in a different place.

Her condition improved rapidly.

Case# 153. Sudden school failure.

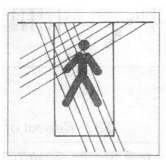

The child had been a very good student.

She then moved to another house just before junior high school.

Beginning at that time, she had headaches and frequent nosebleeds.

No one paid much attention to these symptoms.

However, her family became very upset when the girl suddenly failed in school.

She had to repeat a grade.

I thought that the real reason for the bad grades might be an undiagnosed and unrecognized illness, caused by zones of disturbance.

I urged the parents to seek medical advice. The doctor found abscesses in the sinus cavity.

The bed was moved and the patient responded favourably to treatment.

Case# 1430. After her father's untimely death,

(cancer of the pancreas), Christine was allowed to sleep in her father's bed.

She immediately became ill, suffered from insomnia, restlessness and lack of concentration and threw up frequently.

She failed in school and had to repeat her grade.

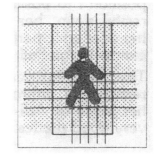

The bed was moved and three weeks later I learned by letter that Christine was sleeping well.

Later I was informed that her grades in school had improved again.

Case# 251. The most forgetful child in her class.

M., age 10, slept above 'pulling water'.

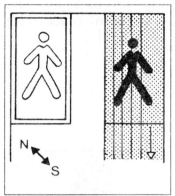

When she got up in the morning, she often felt so dizzy that she fell back into bed.

Her skin looked sallow, she had stomach aches most of the time, was very tired, could not concentrate or remember things and did very poorly in school.

Most of these symptoms improved or disappeared once her bed was moved.

Case# 237. Repeat of entrance exams for junior high.

M., at 12 years of age, was the smallest and least developed child in her grade.

She was restless, nervous, slow and forgetful and did very poorly in school.

Her bed was moved by coincidence (from position I to position II).

From that time on, she enjoyed restful sleep, her appetite improved, she felt better and her academic performance improved.

She did well in her exams in the Fall.

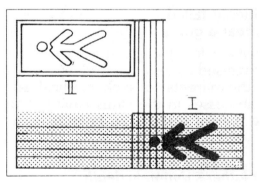

The following year she surprised her teachers with her remarkable improvement in her physical development, her sense of well-being and self-confidence, and with her very good grades.

Case# 162. Was she playing truant ?

This very sensitive girl woke every morning with pains in various parts of her body and felt unable to go to school.

She was also very pale, tired and did not want to eat.

During the day she recovered somewhat and in the afternoon she wanted to go outside to get some fresh air.

Thus the suspicion arose that she was avoiding school.

She had missed school frequently and was unable to catch up with the rest of her class.

Her grades were unsatisfactory, despite her intelligence.

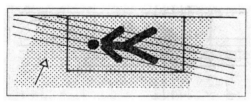

She had to repeat a grade twice.

After the bed was moved, she recovered completely.

Case# 1251c. He stopped growing and failed in school.

This 13 year old boy looked like a 10-year-old.

Norbert had slept for three years on the same spot.

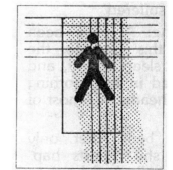

During that time he did not grow an inch, and did not gain a pound.

He could not fall asleep at night and felt extremely tired in the morning.

His scholastic achievements were poor.

However, as soon as the bed was moved, he was able to go to sleep and he felt better.

His grades improved dramatically.

One of his teachers commented on how interested and motivated he had suddenly become.

He gained 8 pounds and grew an inch within a month.

His father felt that a miracle had been performed.

Case# 1036. This 10-year-old felt desperate.

She had been sleeping above a double crossing for seven years.

During that time she suffered from nightmares, cried out in her sleep, had fevers all the time, suffered from stomach aches and lacked appetite.

She looked emaciated, had no energy or enthusiasm, even though her parents and siblings were affectionate and patient with her.

She could not pay attention to her schoolwork, fell asleep in school, and finally even refused to go to school.

Medical and psychological treatment brought no improvement.

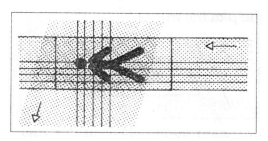

Only after the bed was moved could she recuperate, and finally her health was restored.

Case# 264. Shivering in bed.

Anita, at 10 years old, was very pale and sick a lot.

Her schoolwork suffered. She told me:

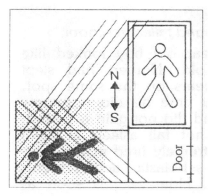

"I have been sleeping in this room for the past year. I sleep poorly, and I am so tired in the morning and I have headaches most of the time".

Change of bed !

After only three days she reports happily:

"Now I sleep very well and feel well. And I am so happy, because I am finally warm in bed. Before my bed was moved, I was always so cold in bed".

Case# 654. 9-year-old girl - a spinal fracture in a skiing accident.

The leg did not heal for a full year.

Her physician recommended that the house be examined since he knew from experience that the healing process was slowed down in the presence of zones of interference.

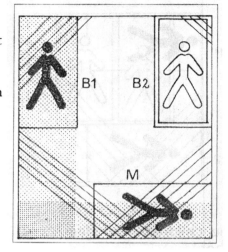

The girl was put into a room which was free of harmful rays, and slowly she began to mend.

Brother No.1 woke every morning clammy from perspiration.

He was put in a bunk-bed above brother No.2.

He felt better immediately.

Brother No.2 always felt well and slept well.

Case# 164. After her grandfather's death

(he had died six months earlier from lung cancer),

Lotte was given the privilege of sleeping in her grandfather's old bed.

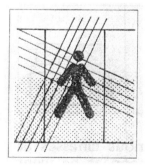

She immediately lost her appetite, suffered from headaches, had trouble sleeping and lost many days from school.

As soon as the bed was moved to another location, she felt better again.

Case# 881 b. Schoolchildren in Argentina

Boy No.1, 7 years old, sleeps restlessly and climbs into his brother's bed almost every night, without fully awakening.

Boy No.2 sleeps well and is healthy.

Girl No.1 (M1) sleeps well and is healthy.

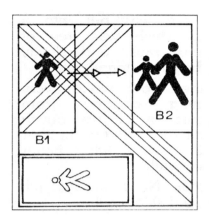
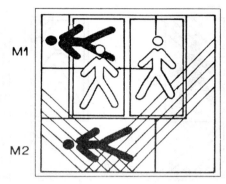

Girl No.2 (M2) slept here for two years and had academic problems during that time.

The beds were moved, and I was informed by letter that the children now sleep well and perform much better in school

Case# 1176c. The most troublesome child in the classroom

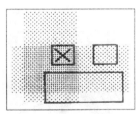

had her desk above a water crossing.

She was nervous, fidgety, disruptive, and could not pay attention in class.

After she was moved to another place in the classroom, her behaviour improved markedly.

Case# 325. Gus, 10 years old, had many serious illnesses at home, especially kidney infections.

As soon as he went to the boarding school, his health improved, presumably because he slept in an area free of rays.

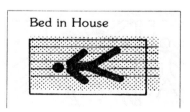

Bed in House

Case# 1506. Irene, 12 years old,

had been well at home and I assume that she slept in a place free of harmful rays.

But in the boarding school her sleep patterns were disturbed, she suffered from chronic bronchitis, and in general her well-being suffered.

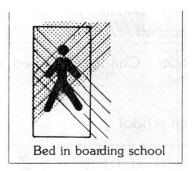

Bed in boarding school

After the bed was moved in the boarding school, her health improved.

Case# 134. Epileptic attacks ?

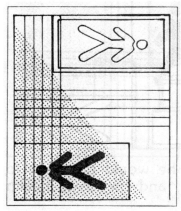

Ingrid had always been a good student.

18 months ago the family moved and since then she has had headaches, trouble concentrating, and poor school performance.

She had three attacks which looked like epilepsy.

She was hospitalized and put on heavy medication.

The attacks stopped, but the headaches continued.

After 6 months I was asked to examine the apartment.

The bed was moved and the headaches subsided.

The neurologist, according to the mother, was very surprised to find such unexpected improvement.

Her school performance, too, has improved.

Case# 268 "Just imagine all the pain !"

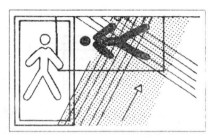

"Every morning something else bothers you.

You just want to get out of going to school."

The mother of an 8-year-old child could not understand how the child could complain of different pains all the time.

The examination of the apartment solved the problem.

Bladder infection, Kidney infection, Sleep disturbances, Poor grades, Repeating a grade.

Change of bed; improvement after a very short time.

Case# 327. A senior in high school

had his bed as well as his desk at home above a zone of disturbance.

His family had lived in the house for 18 months, and during that time the boy had not felt well.

He suffered constantly from headaches, could not bring himself to concentrate on his studies, and asked for painkillers.

His mother refused and reproached him for making it all up so that he would not have to study.

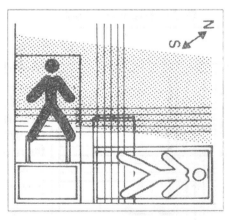

The furniture was moved, and the boy's health returned.

Case# 519. Classroom in a school in Hallein

This is where a girl fainted twice. She also missed school frequently.

"I always had a backache when I spent too much time at the desk."

Recommendation:

'Rotating classroom':

The children should be moved to a different spot every three weeks so that no child has the disadvantage of spending a year above a zone of disturbance.

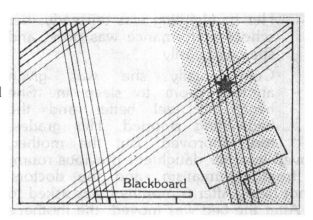

Blackboard

Case# 1247. The negative comment on the report card

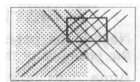

was that the student did not actively participate in the classroom.

But her desk had been directly above a zone of disturbance.

Case# 1031. Confused, absentminded, and two fainting spells.

That was what happened to student S.

He, too, had his desk above a zone of disturbance.

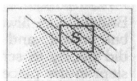

Case# 403. She had a crying spell almost every day.

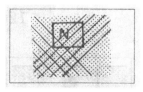

She and two other children had their desks moved, and the symptoms of all three children disappeared.

<u>Case# 120. Because she was a bed wetter</u> the 13 year old was not allowed to go along on the ski vacation.

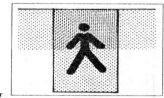

She had been nervous ever since she had been very little, and never stopped wetting the bed.

Her handwriting was unsteady, her school performance was poor, and she cried easily.

Coincidentally she was given another room to sleep in. She began to feel better and the bedwetting stopped.   Her grades, too, improved.

But the mother, who now had moved into her daughter's previous room, began to suffer from rheumatism, and the doctors' prescriptions did not help.

After 6 months I was asked to assess the house.

After the bed was moved, the mother's condition improved

Case# 542. "Why aren't you like your sister ?"

Neither the parents nor the teachers had an inkling why the younger of the two sisters had so many problems.

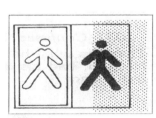

Anna was always healthy, good-humoured, and energetic. She did well in school.

Bridget was always tired, often in a bad mood, and frequently sick, and did poorly in school.

The two sisters slept in the places indicated for many years.

<u>Case# 1264. 16-year-old high school student</u>

H, slept in this location for two years.

During that time she had insomnia, fatigue, trouble concentrating, stomach aches, depression, and poor school achievement.

She flunked all of her finals.

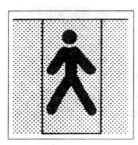

She was called 'lazy' by her teachers, despite the fact that she spent much time in front of her books.

She had problems remembering facts.

The bed was moved, and after 2 months I was informed by letter that the listlessness and frequent depression were gone, and that her enthusiasm for school and for learning had come back.

Case# 1049. A student in Linz

woke up in the morning in a bad mood, and had trouble waking up.

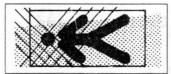

He had frequent colds. His aunt, who had slept in the same place previously, but in the opposite direction, had pains in her legs.

The bed was moved to another spot and soon I was informed by letter that his mood had changed for the better and that his health had definitely improved.

Case# 1301. A nursing student had severe headaches

ever since she began sleeping in her dormitory bed.

She also felt tired, and suffered from a sore throat.

Only after the bed was moved could the doctor's efforts bring results.

Case# 629. A college student

(18 years old) rented a room near the university. Thereafter she suffered from stomach aches every morning, and frequently from headaches also.

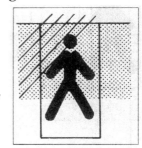

Soon after she moved her bed I heard from her that she now slept well, and felt well, and also that she shuddered to think that she might have slept in the same spot for the next 5 years.

The woman who had occupied the room before her had been studying to be a teacher.

She had been ill for the two years she had been there, and was forced to give up her plans to be a teacher.

Case# 1340. The 'eternal' student, 35 years old.

Despite his intelligence and his diligence, he did poorly in his exams.

He suffered from tiredness, lack of concentration, and kidney problems; he had surgery for kidney stones.

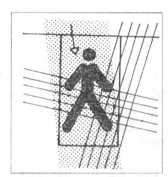

Despite his preparation, he became frozen with anxiety before every test.

He finally completed his studies at age 35.

A week afterwards I examined his apartment.

He moved to a different location and has done well and felt well ever since.

3. Case Studies of Teachers, Professors and Principals

Case# 1299. The teacher, Mr. F.,

suffered from a severe nervous disorder, shaking palsy.

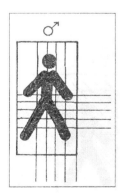

He had several stays in a psychiatric hospital, several leaves of absence.

Medical science could not help.

He took early retirement.

Changing the position of the bed brought relief, but not recovery.

Case# 477. A young female teacher

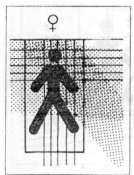

had lived in the same apartment for the past 18 months.

During that time she had not been feeling well, with symptoms of compulsion neurosis.

(A double crossing was found.)

Doctors could not help, nor could hospitalizations or sick leaves.

Only after the bed was moved to another place did the physician and psychiatrist become effective with their treatment.

Case# 1341. A young teacher - severe rheumatism.

She had lived in her apartment for the past seven years, and had been ill during all that time with severe rheumatism.

She had taken sick leave for the past nine months. A quote from her letter:

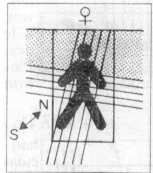

"I was totally exhausted and depressed, because I had not been able to sleep for the past year.

Since we moved the bed around, I feel infinitely better, have no trouble sleeping, and I was able to go back to work after five weeks."

Case# 1042. A teacher and his wife.

At first the husband slept at position No. 1, and he became very ill with rheumatism. His wife slept at position No. 2, and was well.

A draft from the window was suspected as the cause of the illness, and thus the couple exchanged places, since the woman seemed more healthy.

Now the man slept at the edge of the bed and soon recovered.

The woman became ill with rheumatism and neuritis within a very short time.

The bed was then moved and the woman wrote:

"Everything is much better - blood pressure and the neuritis.

We are so grateful for what you have done for us.

I don't think I could have gone on much longer".

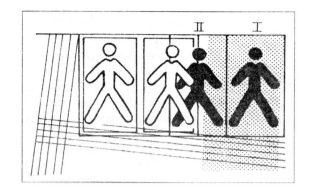

Case# 841. Help came too late

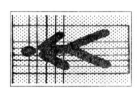

but there was some relief after the bed was moved after 51 years.

Mrs. D., a former classmate, was chronically ill, despite the best medical care available.

Pleurisy, hoarseness, died at 52 years from lung cancer.

Case# 487. Dr. A., a professor of religion,

had sleeping problems, heart and circulatory disease.

After a change of bed position, he wrote:

"Since I moved my bed, I feel so much better and more energetic, and I also can sleep well at night".

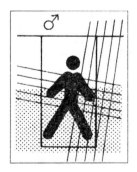

Case# 1293b. Dr. M., Professor of biology.

Since sleeping for 18 months in the same bed, she suffered from polyarthritis.

The doctor recommended that the bed be moved to a different place.

After seven weeks, I received a letter:

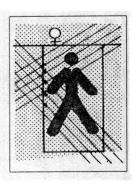

"I noticed very soon a significant change for the better in my condition. I wake up alert and refreshed.

My neck and shoulders are completely free of pain, and the previous tension is gone.

For the past three weeks, I can also move my knees again. I am literally another person!"

Case# 157. "I nearly went out of my mind"

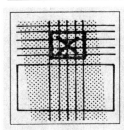

"I was unable to concentrate, I had headaches, stomach aches, nausea, and could not eat. I had to postpone my exams".

This report came from a teacher.

Later on, while located at a place free of radiation, he was able to pass his tests.

Case# 1096b. Standing above disturbance zones while teaching.

A teacher in Salzburg had coughing spells, loss of voice, abdominal and back pains, exhaustion, and sick leave.

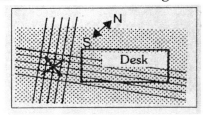

Case# 27. Principal of a secondary school in Salzburg.

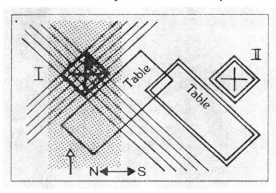

Place I: Lack of concentration, nervousness, many different physical complaints, frequent sick leave.

(Felt well outside the school building.)

Early retirement.

His successor became tired after a short time.

Place II: Repositioning of furniture; feeling of well-being.

Case# 1351. Three high school principals.

They had their office chairs above disturbance zones in Place I:

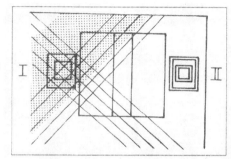

Principal A (1958 - 1968): two heart attacks.

Principal B (1969 - 1973): nervous break down.

Principal C (1973 - 1974): complains of feeling cold and general lack of good health.   The furniture was moved at once.

Then I learned that a former principal (1954 - 1958) had been in place II and had been in the best of health.

Principal C wrote to me that once his chair was moved to place II, he no longer suffered from feeling cold and that his health is very good now.

Case# 1380. University of Salzburg.

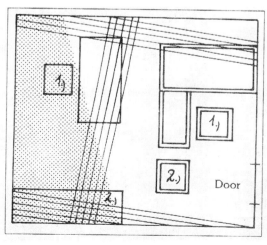

The Department of Philosophy, lecture room and examination room.

1. the lecturer.

2. for the students.

Examination of the locations of the furniture led to re-arrangements as shown in the diagram, to assure a better change for successful test-taking by the students.

8

Case# 743. Workspace of Professor Paul Weingartner,

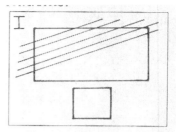

in his apartment in Salzburg.

Feeling of well-being, high energy, even in the evenings.

Adjacent room: increasing feeling of not being up to par, and after 30 minute he felt unable to continue working.

He suspected cooking fat to be the cause of the discomfort.

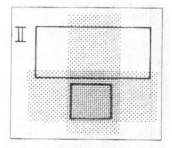

Also suspected an illness of some kind.

Six weeks later he moved to place III with an accompanying sense of well-being.

An examination of the apartment was conducted.

He returned to place I, feels well again, and is able to work productively and with concentration.

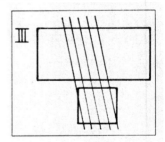

Dr. Paul Weingartner confirms the correctness of this report.

4. Factual and Statistical Information

About Different Areas of Medicine

A: Neurology

(Diseases of the brain, nervous disorders, and emotional disorders.)

A team of physicians and psychologists, under the leadership of Professor Gerhart Harrer, M.D., medical director of the Psychiatric Hospital in Salzburg, and Professor Wilhelm Revers, director of the Psychology, Department at the University of Salzburg, write in their article 'Music and the Vegetative Nervous System' (Ciba-geigy, Basel):

"We see a frantic development of newer and better diagnostic and therapeutic methods.

Nevertheless, the number of patients who are sent home with an explanation like 'this is only in your imagination' or 'its just your nerves' by their doctors has actually increased.

And yet, such a diagnosis can hardly be satisfactory to the physicians, let alone the patients."

How right these doctors and psychologists are.

And those unfortunate people who have been exposed to zones of disturbance are the ones who have to hear these sad statements the most !

How much longer will this have to go on ?

Perhaps not too long anymore, since more and more doctors are beginning to pay attention to the importance of disturbance zones, and to recommend that their patients change the location of their bed on a trial basis for a few weeks or months.

Also, they encourage their patients to pay attention to the places in which they feel well.

Professor Erwin Ringel, M.D. (Vienna), a well-known and successful psychiatrist in whom patients have the utmost confidence, invited me to speak about the results of my research during the Salzburg University Week in 1975.

I spoke about the fact that in all cases of depression that had come to my attention (by that time it was 124 cases), a strong geopathic disturbance zone had been present underneath the sleeping area.

Dr. Ringel replied in the public discussion:

"I am convinced that disturbance zones can have a damaging effect on people. But as far as endogenous depression is concerned, I know that the cause is a metabolic disease."

No doubt Dr. Ringel is right. Metabolic diseases are inducing the depression.

But as to the basis, the unrecognized cause 'in the background', one has to look at the disturbance zones.

For I need to mention that I found zones of disturbance with as many as 276 people suffering from metabolic diseases - as a matter of fact, I never saw a person with a metabolic disorder where disturbance zones had not been present.

Therefore, it is a fact that our observations are not mutually exclusive, but rather that both statements are true and justified.

Dr. Lothar von Kolitscher, M.D., has been able to explain both by a common denominator, by stressing the fact that disturbance zones weaken a person's resistance to disease.

I would like to quote just one of the many witnesses, a young Swiss woman (Case# 1696), who proved again that depressions can indeed be reduced by a change of position of the bed.

She had consulted many doctors, because of exhaustion, severe depressions, dizziness, nervous heart conditions, and many other complaints which had gone on for years.

She asked me to investigate their apartment.

Her bed, as is the case for most severely chronically ill patients, stood directly above a water and curry crossing.

Within six weeks she wrote:

"I am just fine !

Since we moved the beds, I sleep well and my depressions have lessened considerably.

Our little boy also sleeps much better..."

The majority of people react to geopathic zones with sleep disturbances.

Some have trouble falling asleep at night, others suffer from nightmares, or toss and turn restlessly for hours, and some have a deep, almost narcoleptic sleep.

All of them are tired in the morning, discouraged, and physically and mentally exhausted.

And yet, no one will take issue with the fact that a restful and deep sleep is essential for the daily recuperation of a person, and especially necessary for the maintenance of emotional health and equilibrium.

The use of sleeping pills to achieve sleep is not the same as a normal and undisturbed deep sleep, as everyone will agree.

And yet, how many people resort to sleeping pills night after night, just so they can sleep at all.

I often hear from people after they no longer sleep above a zone of disturbance:

"Now I don't have to use sleeping pills anymore."

Constant lack of sleep has consequences, ranging from nervousness to neuroses, depression, irritability, and hostility.

I have had the opportunity to observe people who did not seem to suffer from physical ailments, but who became emotionally ill.

They were at odds with themselves and with 'all the world' around them.

One mother wrote to me about such a state her child had been in, and about how much better her child was doing since the bed had been moved.

Another mother introduced me to her two-and-a-half year old child. I was taken aback by the 'mean' look this child had.

The mother complained to me that she was at her wit's end, because the child was so hard to handle.

She had another child who was easy to get along with and easy to take care of.

She said she did her best to be fair and patient, and yet it did not seem to make any difference to the behaviour of the younger child.

The following picture evolved from the examination of the sleeping places:

Child A slept directly above a zone of disturbance crossing.

His sleep was fitful, he fell out of bed frequently, and woke up in a bad mood and very tired.

Child B slept soundly in his un-radiated little bed, and woke up in the morning happy and full of energy.

A week later I met the mother, who reported happily:

"The whole of last week (Child A) slept beautifully and he is the best little boy imaginable. His whole behaviour has changed."

A third case of severe emotional illness:

An intelligent 12 year old girl woke up every morning full of hostility and hatred towards her 'unsympathetic' mother, who made her get up, even though she was still 'sooooo tired', and she felt so weak and so miserable.

Then she expressed envy toward her baby sister, who was allowed to sleep as much as she wanted and who was taken care of by the mother.

The sleeping place of this 12 year old girl was located above three subterranean water currents and a Curry strip.

The emotional illness of a child is often not recognized as such; and thus the cause for those disorders is not often looked for.

There is a prevalent opinion that such children have to be taught to behave by punishment and discipline.

Some other parents tend simply to ignore such a child.

What is really called for is to take care of such a child with as much love and devotion as is being lavished on a physically sick child.

To be punished is perceived by such an emotionally sick child as an act of gross injustice.

A child like this can become bitter, and continue with that attitude for the rest of his life, while a feeling of acceptance and belonging would diminish the suffering and assist the recovery.

You can imagine how deeply affected I was when I discovered that disturbance zones are the cause of so many family tragedies brought on by the constant ill-humour of people; or again, when I could point to disturbance crossings in cases of long-term hostility, envy, and hatred among people.

Many people suffering from geopathic effects have a tendency to blame their fellow men for their discomfort.

The same is true for couples who suffer from those effects.

A reputable Viennese attorney, himself a dowser, made the same observation over and over again, that 'those couples', already on the way to a divorce, began to handle their differences and forgive one another as soon as they relocated to a radiation-free spot.

I too had the good fortune several times to witness the resurgence of strength and emotional integrity leading to a reconciliation, as soon as the people were removed from the damaging influence of the various earth rays.

Yet despite these comments - despite the certainty that many times the real cause can be found in the disturbance zones - I have no doubt that people sometimes make wrong decisions in their lives.

Those decisions have to do with choosing egotism instead of love, domination instead of compassion, and retaliation instead of forgiveness.

Many people do not become bitter and hard through their experience of illness and suffering, but instead more tolerant, more understanding and compassionate, and more mature.

However, that does not give us the right to keep other people suffering, as long as we have a way to help them.

But now back to the research.

My statistical data were compiled in 1974. The research material up to that point amounted to exactly 1,500 investigations of apartments and houses. The data were tabulated over the course of several weeks, with great attention to detail.

From about 300 entries, the different specialties of medicine were statistically compiled.

Thus, every physician can inform himself of the fact that earth influences do not just play a minor role, but they make a significant contribution as the cause of illnesses.

The examples in the following sections are drawn from material collected from the first 1,500 examinations of apartments.

Case# 18. Compulsive crying and suicidal thoughts.

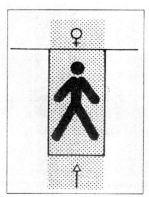

Mrs.H., a former student of mine, is happily married.

'Without any reason' she experienced crying spells every evening, suffered from nightmares, and was haunted by severe suicidal thoughts: Cause: 'Pushing water'.

The bed was relocated. It took eight days for her to sleep and feel better. (It is not unusual for some people to take a few days, even weeks to feel better.)

In her letter, she writes:

"I cannot tell you how different I feel and how happy I am now."

Case# 1087. Waking up in a daze.

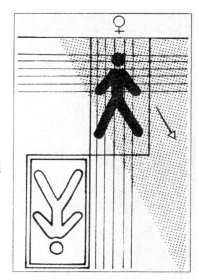

This woman 'blacks out' frequently (lack of adequate blood supply to the head.) This was caused by 'pulling water'.

I was asked by her general practitioner to see this woman after he heard one of my lectures. He had seen her as a patient, rather unsuccessfully, for the past 20 years.

The woman suffered from chronic headaches, frequent pains in the heart area, constant abdominal pains, vomiting, and had had several operations.

Eight days after I saw her, I received a postcard:

"We moved the bed arid I feel so much better."

Case# 81. Migraine

The couple lived in a room for 18 months.

During that time, they were ill.

He felt constantly 'under the weather'.

She suffered from severe migraines, insomnia, and many other complaints.

A letter from them reported rapid improvement as soon as their bed was moved to another place.

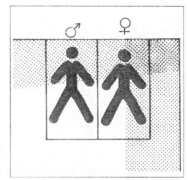

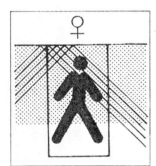

Case# 1354. Cerebral apoplexy

Piercing pain at the back of the head.

Migraine, cramps, low blood pressure, anxieties.

Change of sleeping place recommended.

Case# 787. Television close to the bed, built into the closet.

Professor P. had slept for the past three years on the same spot.

During that time, he suffered from abdominal distress, despite an appropriate diet

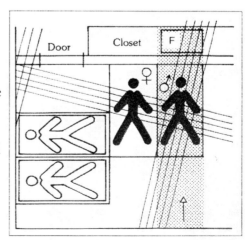

For the past six months, he had a television set behind the wall and during that time had suffered from 'unbearable' headaches every night - televisions emit reflected radiation.

The bed was moved immediately.

Two weeks later he wrote in a letter:

"I feel just fine. No more pains and I feel well and energetic..."

Case# 1229. A young couple in Salzburg,

lived for four years in their apartment, with much physical discomfort.

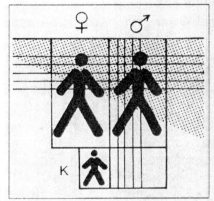

He suffered from insomnia, a feeling of pressure around the chest, as though 'run over by a bulldozer', convulsive vomiting in the mornings, severe depressions.

He had been hospitalized in a psychiatric clinic.

Their child refused to stay in his father's bed, and in his own bed he slept on the very edge.

The mother had been diagnosed as having breast nodules.

Immediate change of beds.

Instantaneous recovery.

Case# 1315. Four neurologists were unable to help.

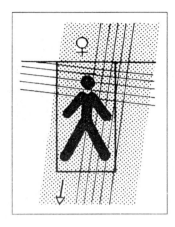

A further report by the same woman:

"I always felt well as a young girl.

I got married ten years ago.

We moved into this house and I have been sick ever since."

Nightmares, always tired, nervous, shaking in bed, severe headaches, and severe depressions.

The four neurologists I consulted could not provide any relief. I was desperate.

Then I decided to travel to Linz to Dr. Polzer, hoping that he could help.

"He advised me to move my bed, because only then can any kind of treatment be successful."

Case# 300. Neurasthenia also called weak nerves,

was the diagnosis. Yet, Mr. N. suffered from severe pains.

I felt so sorry for him.

Eight specialists could not find the real illness.

This was told to me by a sympathetic and experienced country doctor.

While on sick leave, Mr. N. was lying in the living room on the couch and the pains became unbearable.

The furniture was re-arranged, and improvement was instantaneous.

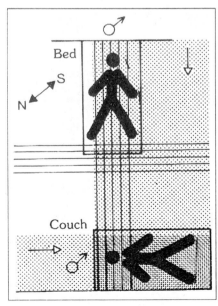

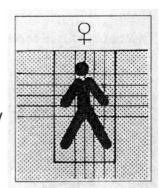

Case# 1140. "It is only hysteria !"

"That is my husband's opinion, and to him that means imagination and bad temper.

And yet I hurt so much everywhere, especially at night in bed; I have heart, gall bladder, and kidney ailments, gout and rheumatism.

I had a thyroidectomy. But any time I sleep in the other room I feel so much better". Recommendations: Move the bed !

Case# 1438c. Mrs. T. lay unconscious for two days

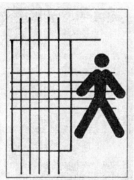

on the floor next to her bed. Her daughter found her in time for her life to be saved.

Mrs. T. could not recall anything. What was the cause ? Ever since she had moved into that apartment, she suffered from insomnia and a general 'not well feeling'.

On the 10th floor, exactly above her, Professor C. used to have his bed.

He suffered from a nervous stomach and intestinal discomfort.

Everything became much better for Mrs, T. as soon as her bed was moved.

Case# 894. Psychological agitation

to a high degree was the diagnosis for Mrs C. in Argentina.

Her physician asked me for a consultation. He felt that she was his most difficult case.

These people had lived in a shack for 20 years.

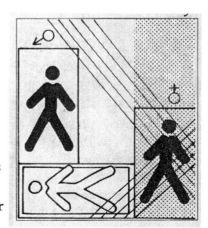

The woman had been ill all that time.

Lately she had begun screaming with pain all night long.

Her husband was always well.

After the bed was moved, the woman calmed down and felt better.

Case# 745. Why did a divorce take place ?

A physician asked me to see his most difficult patient.

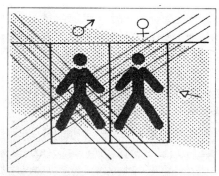

The woman said:

"My husband was aggressive and always in a bad mood.

He asked for the divorce. I have terrible pain all over my body, severe depressions, and a nervous disorder."

In many cases of alcoholism or marital discord I have found the fundamental cause to be the crossing of zones of disturbance.

Case# 491. Cerebral Aneurysm

The man is healthy; the woman died at a young age.

The man reports:

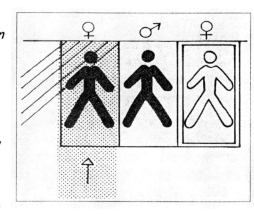

"My first wife was always in good health. But at night she suffered from headaches.

Suddenly she had an aneurysm and died eight days later. Now my second wife, too, suffers from headaches at night."

After moving the bed: well-being !

Considering the state of medical science today, we have to assume the presence of strong zones of disturbance whenever somebody dies young.

Therefore I recommend an examination of the house or apartment, before a remarriage.

Case# 1438b. Encephalitis

A young mother who was a nurse by profession reported:

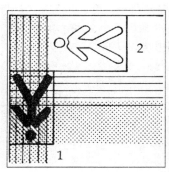

"When he was only two years old, my child used to sleep above this double crossing. He tossed and turned at night. He contracted encephalitis, tonsilitis, mumps on both sides, as well as pneumonia.

He was hospitalized for 8 weeks.

Fortunately, I moved the child's bed at that time. Since then he has slept well and feels well."

Case# 862. Spastic Torticollis

Mrs. D. had her head above a double crossing: WxWxCxC.

In such cases, a cure is impossible.

She reported:

"I have terrible headaches, especially at night. I also have sciatica, and it hurts so much more during the night.

I have consulted so many doctors. I spent 40 days in the hospital for nervous disorders in Salzburg; and at the University Hospital in Vienna, one physician recommended brain surgery".

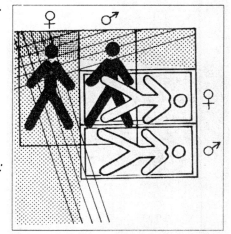

<u>Case# 440. A psychiatrist was convinced</u>

that his patient had guilt feelings, and was annoyed that Mrs. D. claimed to be free of guilt feelings.

What then caused the years of illness of this secretary from Munich ?

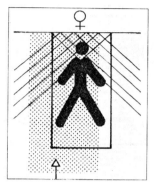

'Pushing water' and a Curry crossing.

This resulted in total exhaustion in the morning, swollen eyelids for many hours, headaches, forgetfulness, depressions, abdominal cramps, and numb fingers.

It was all too much for her.

The doctors could not help, and her illness became worse.

I recommended that the bed be moved.

<u>Case# 121. Inflammation of cranial nerves four times</u>

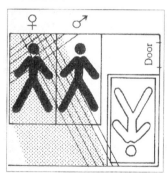

I frequently met an old lady who usually complained:

"Today I have such terrible headaches again.

I have had inflammation of a nerve in my head four times and had to go to the hospital every time."

She asked me to come to her house. Her husband had died of cancer.

I recommended that the bed be moved to a different place, and I offered to help her with it.

She refused, because she was worried about how the room would look. About six months later I inquired whether she had rearranged the room. She replied:

"No, a neighbour of mine said that all of those things are sheer nonsense."

He who cannot accept advice cannot be helped !

Case# 1496. Alcoholism becomes evident

in many cases only after the person has slept above crossed zones of disturbance.

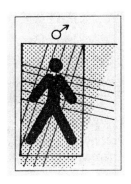

The alcohol serves the purpose of masking the constant sense of 'not feeling well'.

This was true of Mr. N. He eventually died of cancer of the larynx.

Case# 1484. Trigeminal Neuralgia

In 1958, a man moved into a new apartment and became ill almost immediately.

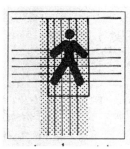

In the morning he suffered from pains 'from head to foot', especially in the lower back.

He had three trigeminus operations for neuralgia: in 1959 in Bad Ischl, in 1960 in Innsbruck, and in 1963 in Graz.

Moving the bed at first brought very little relief, but later there was marked improvement, and finally almost complete recovery.

Case# 510. Cramps in the legs

Mrs. R. suffered from cramps in the legs almost every night, and also from insomnia, duodenal ulcer, and phlebitis.

Four months after moving her bed, Mrs. R. Wrote:

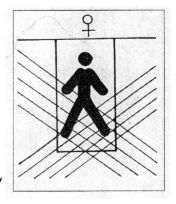

"What a blessing to be able to sleep through the night.

Ever since I rearranged the bed, I have had neither pains nor cramps in the legs."

Case# 1254. A nurse reports:

I am now sleeping on the new location that you recommended.

I sleep very well indeed.

The chills and the pins and needles in my feet have disappeared completely.

Case# 987. Mr. H. has multiple sclerosis.

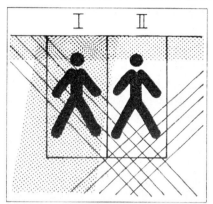

Mrs. H. from Salzburg asked for an examination.

After wards I asked her which bed her husband was sleeping in.

She said: *"In this one,"* and pointed to bed No. II.

I looked surprised and she explained that he had been sleeping in bed No. I for 7 years and that they had changed beds only two weeks ago.

I recommended that both beds be moved to a different place.

Case# 456. The best physician cannot help

as long as the patient lies over a double crossing.

The first wife could not stand it; she left him and later divorced him.

The second wife was desperate. The doctor asked me to examine the bedroom.

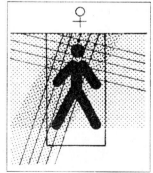

The woman had sleep disturbances, 'terrible' headaches, nervous disorders (hospitalized), heart disease (very elevated heart rate in bed), gallbladder dysfunction, kidney stones, oedema.

The bed was moved immediately, and the doctor was then effective with his treatment.

One page from the Statistical Summary:

<u>Nervous disorders, Depression, Hospitalizations</u>

Entry No.	Case No.	Geopathic Conditions	Symptoms
111	1121	W CxC	Often very discouraged.
112	1137	WxW CxC	Very discouraged at night in bed, 'would like to run away'.
113	1137c	CxC	Psychiatric hospital.
114	1140	W CxC	Supposedly 'hysterical'.
115	1144	W CxC	Very despondent.
116	1148b	CxC	Nervousness.
117	1150	Pushing WxC	Severe depression, seriously suicidal.
118	1156	Cold CxC W	Anxiety, shaking, and crying spells.
119	1177	WxW C	Nervousness, depressions.
120	1178	WxW C	Nervous disorders, depressions.

Summary statistics for cases 1 - 1500 for neurological problems:

Influences from the earth in 349 people with severe sleep disorders and nightmares, and in 289 people with headaches and brain diseases.

Some people gave more accurate information about their symptoms:
   9: Migraine.
  14: Drowsiness and dizziness in the morning.
   3: Stabbing pains at the back of the head.
   2: Neuralgia.
  13: Sinusitis.
   9: Meningitis.
   1: Encephalitis.
  15: Seizures and attacks resembling epilepsy.
   1: Trigeminal neuralgia.
   2: Haematoma.
   4: Cerebral tumour.

And geopathic effects on 232 people with nervous disorders and emotional illness like 'nervous-ness', spasms and neuritis, trembling, shaking palsy (6), despondence, irritation and aggression, anxiety (wanting to run away), crying spells, melancholia, depressions (124), to the point of desperation and serious suicidal thoughts (4).

Geopathic effects in 122 people with cramps in the arms and hands, legs and feet (9). Also varicose veins, phlebitis, and open sores on feet and legs (9), thromboses.

Geopathic effects on 23 people who reported that they had to enter a psychiatric clinic for examination or treatment.

Especially strong influences from the search on 144 seriously ill people with a total collapse who could not be helped by any doctor they consulted.

Of these people, 33 slept over a double crossing (WxW x CxC).

No physician, psychiatrist, or psychologist could help them.

Only after they were relocated to a place free of radiation was medical treatment successful.

Exhaustion, especially in the morning, was reported by 238 patients, who had slept above a disturbance zone.

B. Other Disorders

The following case studies concern: Ophthalmology; Ear, Nose, and Throat; Teeth, Mouth, and Diseases of the Jaw; Patients with Focal Infection; Dermatology; Orthopaedics; Pulmonary Diseases; Internal Medicine; Urology; Gynaecology; Rheumatoid Diseases.

Case# 902. Bishop C. Rosenhammer

His head rested above a magnetic crossing and a water vein, and he suffered for many years from a serious eye disease, which led to almost complete blindness and many operations, sinus problems, furunculosis on the chin, and chronic bronchitis.

"I feel so much better since I moved my bed. My eyes are getting better, too, and I am so grateful for Käthe Bachler's advice.

Jose C. Rosenhammer, San Ignacio de Velasco, Bolivia."

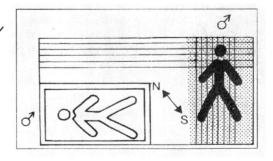

Case# 259. Little Veronica (16 months old)

had frequent high fevers, 102°-102.5°, and sore throats. The physician, Dr. Schaber wrote:

"The family calls me almost every week.

I hospitalized the little girl, and the fever disappeared at once.

The doctors thought that the drug had helped.

After she was dismissed I continued with the medication, but at home it had no effect - her fever started up again almost immediately."

The doctor took me to the house; the bed had to be moved, then fever subsided. The child became well within a very short time.

Case# 1213. Surgery - cancer of the nose,

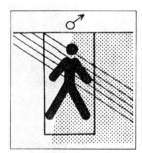

that is what Mr. N. of Innsbruck had to submit to about 10 years ago.

Since he had such a hard time sleeping in his bedroom, he changed rooms after the surgery.

He was fortunate, for that area was found to be free of harmful rays.

Case# 801. Chronic and dangerous nosebleed

was the reason the high school student K. had to go to the hospital several times .

After the bed was moved, she recovered very quickly.

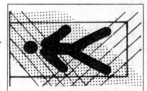

Case# 327. Abscessed teeth,

after moving into a new house 18 months ago (WxC).

Complete healing took place once the bed was moved.

Case# 1325. Strong spasms

in the head area, the neck and the shoulders caused the jaw to move its position so that chewing became difficult.

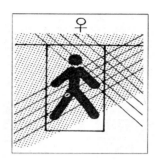

This is what Mrs. N. from Innsbruck reported. The difficulties occurred only after she moved into the present apartment three years ago.

She also suffered from nightmares.

After the bed was moved, she enjoyed more restful sleep and was feeling better in general.

Case3 2386 to 2399.   Patients with Focal Infections.

'Focal Infections' can be lodged in many different areas, but are found most frequently in the roots of teeth and in the jaw.

Dr. Alexander Rossaint, a dentist from Aachen, employs the most modern methods for detecting focal infection, including electro-acupuncture and blood tests.

After reading my book he wondered whether some of those patients with whom he could not achieve a cure were suffering from the influence of the Curry grid.

So he began to use the 'blood drop test' (Dieter Aschoff, M.D. 'Electro-magnetic Blood Test'), which verifies the presence of geopathic zones.

At the same time he asked me to examine the living quarters of those patients.

He did not tell me anything about his own examinations and findings.

Dr. Rossaint wrote very succinctly and clearly about the phenomenon of focal infection in his letter:

"Focal infection points are a constant irritation to the body tissues and often cause undesirable and permanent changes.

This definition was given by Prof. Pischinger, M.D. (Vienna).

In chronic illness, it is wise to consider the possibility of a focal infection in addition to the defined illness.

At the same time we find that chronic illness can be caused by a focal infection.

Focal infections impede the course of any therapy, and it is therefore useful to have a focal infection therapy run concurrent with therapy for a given illness."

Dr. Rossaint accompanied me to the apartments of patients who suffered particularly from focal infection, and he watched me do my work.

He was amazed when he learned that in all cases there was crossing of zones of disturbance above which the patient slept.

(The place of work was examined only if the patient complained of not feeling well during work hours.)

And only then did he tell me that he also had ascertained geopathic interference in all of those patients with the aid of the blood drop test.

Summary of the work on Focal Infection Patients, May 1978

Geopathic Influences

Protocol No.	Patient's Complaint	Sleeping Place	Work Place
2386 Mr. C	"Seriously ill, autonomic nervous disorder which began 5 yrs. ago at his place of work.	WxC	WxC
2387 Mrs. M	Very ill, no doctor can help.	WxWxCxC	
2388 Mrs. W	Quite ill.	WxCxC	
2389 Mrs. H	Chronically ill.	WxC	
2391 Mrs. Ph.	Always exhausted.	WxCxC	
2392 Mr. C	Different ailments.	WxCxC	WxCxC
2395 Mrs. N	Serious nervous disorders, total exhaustion, no organic causes, spent $8000 for treatment.	WxCxC	

2397 AC,DDS	Serious heart ailments for many years, especially pronounced in bed.	WxCxC
2398 Mrs. V	Depression, always tired.	WxCxC
2399 Mrs. C, M.D.	Dizziness, racing heart at night in bed.	WxCxC

Three weeks later I received the following success stories from Dr. Rossaint:

"Some of the cases, 100%. .. some of them 50% (for instance No. 2397, and in such short time ! A very ill dentist had told me:

"No colleague has been able to help me so fast. One of them advised heart surgery for about 30,000 marks but would not guarantee the outcome.

Only the progressive Dr. Rossaint has been able to help his colleague, since he took care of the main culprit ahead of time".

In this same letter, Dr. Rossaint wrote: *"Thanks to your sensitivity you were able to make us aware of such an important issue.*

This issue was apparent at every electro-acupuncture examination I did. You have found with all the examinations of the living places of my patients with focal infection that those people were all suffering from the influence of geopathic disturbances.

Thus we find total concurrence between two independent methods of investigation.

Especially in the case of focal infection we find that the elimination of the stress factors is a precondition before a cure can take place."

Case# 59. Cancer of the tongue

Mrs. N. of Salzburg showed me into an empty room and asked whether there was a 'dangerous area'.

I examined and indicated the 'water crossing'. She said right away:

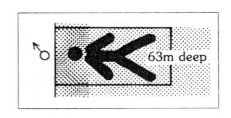

"This is the place where my husband slept. He died of cancer of the tongue".

This very same observation points to the fact that water currents which cross at a point of marked difference in depth (lightning tends to strike there) are particularly strong.

Case# 1358. Cancer of the skin at the left temple

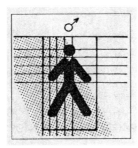

Mr. N. lies on his back.

The edges of a little 'brook' are often particularly strong.

He had surgery and a new place for his bed was recommended

Case# 1260b. Man died of bone cancer at age 45

Here I found a double crossing.

The son reported:

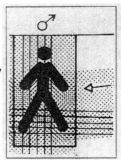

"My father neither drank nor smoked and just the same he was sick so much of the time.

He had to be taken to the hospital since he could not stand it at home in his bed.

Stomach surgery, confined to his bed, bone cancer.

Thirteen years after he moved into this room he died."

Case# 218. Osteomyelitis for several years

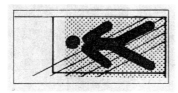

The child was six years old, from Vienna.

After a new place was found for her bed, she recovered very quickly.

<u>Case# 1096. Three generations suffered from severe illnesses.</u>

A family in Tyrol lived in a dank house at the bottom of a mountain.

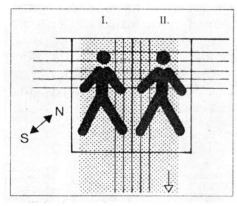

Bed I: Daughter had repeated bouts of meningitis, and chronic bronchitis.

The grandmother had suffered paralysis of the left side for six years.

Bed II: The mother had gallbladder disease, amoebic dysentery, duodenal ulcer, gastritis, anaemia, pancreatic tumour, TB of the spinal column.

The grandfather had been confined to the bed for six years before he died of stomach cancer.

Recommended change of beds, and renewed contact with various physicians.

<u>Case# 1108. Tuberculosis</u>

For ten years, no cure.

Twice an extended stay at a sanatorium for lung diseases.

I received word in a letter that after the bed was moved the patient became well.

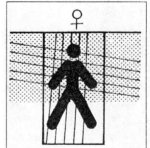

<u>Case# 286. Three generations died of lung cancer,</u>

and all of those people slept in the same bed.

Mrs. N. asked: *"Do you really think that the water veins caused my husband's early death ?"*

Yes, I am sure that a crossing of two zones of disturbance were the main cause of his dying of cancer.

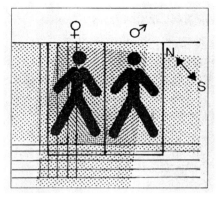

Fact: Water crossings !

Farmer H., his father, and his grandfather, all three of them died at an early age of lung cancer.

Mrs. H. suffered from a malfunctioning gallbladder.

Change of bed brought improvement.

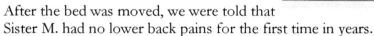

Case# 889. At a German convent in South America.

In the convent Santa Anita, we were told that every nun became sick after just a short time (double crossing was found).

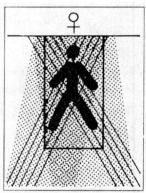

They were affected with ailments of the lungs and liver, pleurisy, rheumatism, deformation of the fingers, heart disease, and sinusitis.

Some of them had to go to the hospital for surgery, and then transferred to another convent where they could get well again.

After the bed was moved, we were told that Sister M. had no lower back pains for the first time in years.

Case# 934. An overdose of digitalis

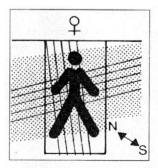

was the case of my little sister Barbara.

She worked as a nurse in the SOS Childrens Village in Cochamba, Bolivia.

The doctor could not understand why none of his medicines helped.

Severe heart ailments, shingles, severe liver and kidney disease.

Unfortunately, my help came too late.

Case# 1214. Severe heart palpitations

She had sleep disturbances, melancholia, nervousness, polyps of the uterus.

Change of bed.   One week later I received a 'thank you' note.

"All of my heart problems are gone !"

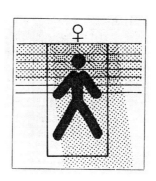

Case# 1106. Cardiac arrest

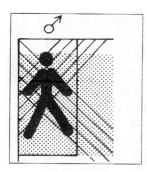

Mr E. was found dead in bed in the morning, without having been ill the night before.

Cardiac arrest was the cause of his death.

He had been sleeping in this bed for only the past two years.

His predecessor Dr. A. also was often ill during the time he slept in this bed.

Pneumonia, abscesses, gallbladder trouble, severe diabetes.

His successor had the apartment examined before he moved in, and moved the bed to a place without any geopathic interference.

He has remained well.

Case# 1443. A physician from Tyrol

took me to his most difficult patient.

He assumed the presence of a zone of disturbance since he could not bring about any improvement in the angina pectoris or in the circulatory problems.

The patient sat during the day on the couch in his daughter's house.

Thus he was exposed to geopathic influences during the day as well as the night.

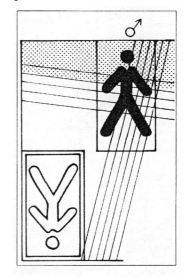

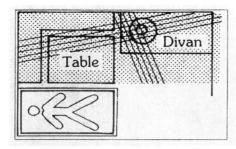

I recommended the purchase of an easy chair to put on a good place and not to use the couch at all anymore.

I received a letter from the physician three months later that the recommendations proved to be 100% successful.

Case# 778. Mrs. L. (Salzburg) had surgery for breast cancer,

kidney stones, and a disc operation.

Her mother had slept in the same bed and had died of a heart attack.

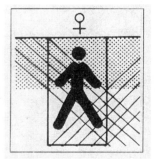

The physician who asked me to examine the apartment told me that the patient recovered soon after she followed my recommendation.

Case# 714. *"My blood sedimentation rate became normal again.*

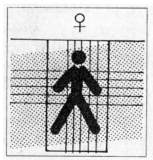

- I am so happy."

This was written to me by a journalist, Mrs. N. , about 6 months after she moved her bed.

Before that she suffered from persistent stomach aches, severe depressions, and a constant feeling of coldness in her bed.

Now she experiences warmth.

Case# 548. *"Finally we found the right medicine !"*

That is what a doctor said, who had no prior knowledge of dowsing.

He did not realize that only after the bed had been put back in its original place could the medicine have a chance to do its work.

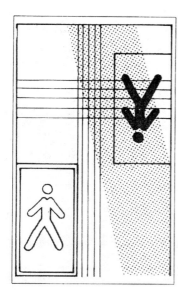

4 year old Sonjâ had been lying for the past 18 months on a zone of disturbance crossing, and she had been very sick the whole time.

Intestinal problems, ear infections, lack of appetite.

No medicine helped.

When I recommended a change of bed, I was told that Sonja slept on that spot for the first 3 years of her life and was always healthy.

She recovered as soon as her bed was moved back to the original spot.

Case# 878. Leukaemia was fatal

For the 16 year old son of a German farmer in Buenos Aires, Argentina.

He had been sleeping above a zone of disturbance crossing.

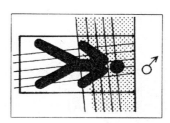

Case# 1397. *"My life was in danger,"*

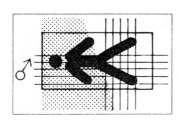

according to the judgement of three physicians.

"A year and a half have passed since I followed your advice and changed my sleeping place, so as to avoid the zones of disturbance which you pointed out to me.

When I asked for your help in May 1974, I had been told by three physicians that I was seriously ill.

I was hardly able to work, and suffered from constant stomach pains.   After I followed your recommendations and sought homeopathic medical care, my condition has changed so dramatically that I feel well and energetic and able to work again."

Case# 565. Stomach cancer

was the cause of death of Mr. L. three years after he moved into this house.

His son's bed is located exactly beneath his on the floor below.

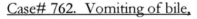

Since moving into this house he too suffers from severe stomach ailments, swelling of the lymph nodes, and abscesses over much of his body.

The doctor had tried to help for years, but to no avail.

A thorough examination in the hospital did not shed light on the disease.

Only after the bed was moved could the medication work and the patient became well.

Case# 762. Vomiting of bile,

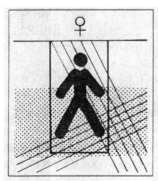

that is what Mrs. I. did every night.

Her husband's grandmother had died of cancer in the same bed.

After she moved her bed, Mrs. I. became well.

Case# 1367. A gall bladder operation

had to be performed on Physician Dr. H.

Ever since she moved to her present sleeping place she had been ill.

She suffered from pain and anxiety attacks at night in bed.

Everywhere else she seemed to sleep well.

She changed the bed immediately and slept better the very first night.

She said:

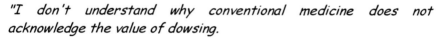

"I don't understand why conventional medicine does not acknowledge the value of dowsing.

It seems to me they ought to be grateful for the help."

Case# 56. Cancer of the liver

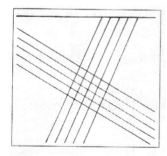

In response to my remark, *"How fortunate that there is no bed above this crossing,"*

I got the answer:

"But the previous owner had his bed at exactly this spot. He died of cancer of the liver."

Case# 1395. Diabetes

A catholic priest suffered for years from sleep disorders and general poor health.

Two and a half months after he moved his bed, he wrote:

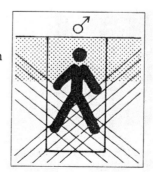

"I am definitely sleeping better and my diabetes is easier to control.

A great relief."

Case# 194. Bleeding from the kidneys

A 20 year old man suffered from bleeding from the kidneys, and also from sleep disorders, colds, and general malaise.

WxCxC was found. The bed was relocated.

His health improved, his sleep improved, he felt better, and eventually became well and energetic.

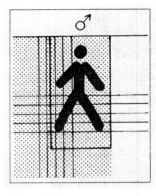

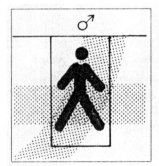

Case# 15. Cancer of the kidneys

was the cause of my brother in law's early death.

He had a tumour as big as two fists.

The crossing of two water veins at 30 metres' difference in depth was also an area for lightning to strike.

Case# 138. Mr. N. had cancer of the bladder.

He slept above a Curry crossing and water veins.

Since the illness had advanced to the last stages already, the changing of the bed brought only slight relief.

Case# 1238. Vegetative Dystonia

Anxiety attacks, palpitations of the heart, deterioration of the discs, very tired in the morning, sore throat, toxaemia at pregnancy, and miscarriage.

Rearrangement of the bed was recommended.

Eight weeks later I received a letter:

"It took quite a long time until I could feel any improvement.

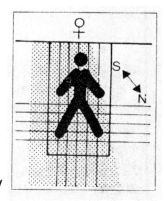

But now I feel much better, I am no longer so tired, no longer have any sore throats, and I feel and look so much better."

Case# 1371. Operation on the colon

Severe abdominal pains for many years.

Two and a half years ago, removal of 40 cm of large intestine, but pain and discomfort persisted, with lack of sleep.

Bed was put in a different place.

Immediately the sleep problems disappeared and the abdominal pains subsided. Felt better in general.

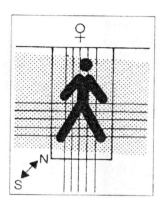

Case# 1458. 'Cancer bed' in a convent in Austria

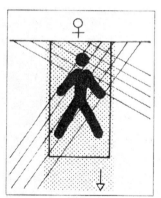

1. Sister M. had a mastectomy.

She was transferred to another room and recovered.

2. Sister F. occupied the same place for the next five years.

She became very ill soon after.

Severe headaches, cerebrospinal meningitis.

After a stay in the hospital she was sent to another convent and recovered.

3. Sister N. had been in this bed for 12 years and was very ill.

She had to undergo three operations for cancer of the colon, and had psoriasis.

The bed was moved and she wrote me a postcard saying that she felt better immediately.

Case# 1356. Mrs. N. wrote the following letter:

"For more than 5 years I have suffered from colitis and consequently from circulatory problems and nervousness.

Repeated stays in hospitals and clinics have not proved ultimately to be effective, since the minute I get home again the old symptoms reappear.

Nobody knows why that is so.

Would it be possible for you to come to my house and conduct an examination ?

It would be an enormous relief for me, if the cause could be ascertained."

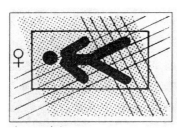

And this shows the result of my examination:

After the bed was moved to a different place, the patient felt better.

Case# 899.   Hospital in El Chochis, Bolivia

Patients are assigned places which are 'free of radiation' so that successful operations are free of later complications 'which could not be explained' (like haemorrhages).

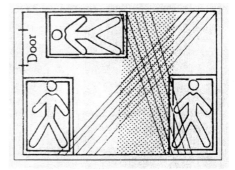

Case# 1136c. Intestinal parasites,

despite treatment and scrupulous attention to hygiene.

Only after Mrs. N. (Salzburg) moved her bed could she recover completely.

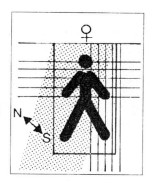

Case# 1251. Dysmenorrhea,

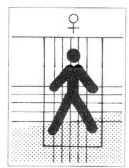

also constant abdominal problems, and infections.

The 17 year old girl moved her bed and wrote to me a month later:

"This time my period was totally free of pain."

Case# 1213. Childlessness

The marriage remained childless for 10 years.

The woman suffered from cramps and intestinal problems.

Only during a vacation, away from their apartment, on the Isle of Rhodes, did she finally get pregnant.

She had a malfunctioning spleen and her kidneys were not working to capacity.

The bed was moved, and there was improvement.

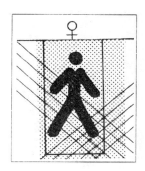

Case# 499. Cysts on both ovaries

Mrs. A. also had marked anemia and heavy menstrual flow.

Her physician requested the examination of the house.

Her husband, a robust looking construction worker, said,

"My health is fine."

As I looked surprised, he added:

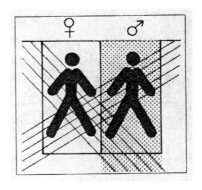

"Oh yes, I had a ruptured appendix and now I suffer alternately from either constipation or diarrhea."

After the bed was moved, both people enjoyed better health.

Case# 624. Cancer of the ovaries

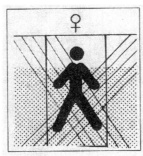

Mrs. L. from Munich had been ill ever since she moved into this house.

Cancer surgery, followed by death.

A letter from the widower said:

".. and just imagine, a boy who sleeps directly beneath her bed on the floor below had a tumour removed from his chest.

And he is only 14 years old."

Case# 281. In Linz:

The first wife died of leukemia at a young age.

The second wife, in the same bed, had toxemic pregnancy, constant headaches and backaches.

A carpenter was called in immediately and the room was rearranged.

A letter advised me of recovery.

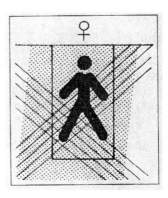

Case# 1071. Alarming weight loss, two miscarriages, no children

That was the state of health of a young Italian woman who had enjoyed good health prior to her marriage.

She had been married for 10 years and in ill health the whole time.

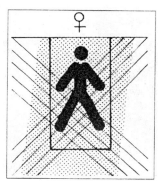

Whenever she sat down on her bed, she got severe pains in her lower back and abdomen, and sometimes also muscle spasms.

She sought help from many physicians, including one at the University Hospital in Innsbruck.

Her physician asked me to see her in Italy since he suspected the influence of zones of disturbance.

After the bed was moved she began to feel better immediately, and she gained 20 pounds the first month.

Case# 583. "Father and mother died at an early age of cancer."

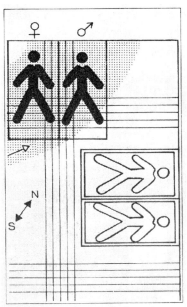

The man died of cancer of the prostate.

His wife died of cancer of the uterus.

The young people said:

"We are sleeping in the same beds, and we, too, always seem to be sick."

Every night, muscle spasms in the legs, pain in the kidney area, exhaustion, severe rheumatism, nervousness.

After I indicated the best place for the beds, I was told that this was also the place where the grandparents had slept, who enjoyed good health and a long life.

The new location of the beds brought about a recovery of the young people within a short period of time.

Case# 942. Gout and rheumatism,

that was what afflicted the director of the Austrian SOS Childrens' Village in Chochamba, Bolivia.

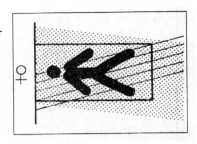

The bed was moved and his health improved dramatically, as written to me in a letter.

Case# 490. Farmer S. suffered from swollen knees.

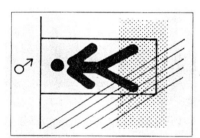

"All by itself, it came on overnight." The bed was moved and he recovered immediately.

Case# 729. Sciatica

A Lutheran minister had slept in the same place for the past four years, suffering from disturbed sleep, pains in the lower back, sciatica and general exhaustion.

He was easily upset.

No physician could find the cause.

Extensive tests and treatments in a hospital setting did not bring the desired results.

But when the bed was moved, he recovered rapidly (letter).

Case# 1304. Attacks of sciatica

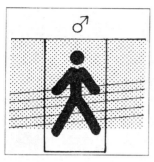

Also heart problems and pain in the lower back.

A physician himself, he could not find any cure.

The bed was moved and he has felt better ever since.

No more sciatica attacks.

Case# 1276. Arthritis, spondylosis

A man from Graz had been suffering from various ailments ever since moving into this bedroom.

He always slept on his back.

He had many complaints, but they always involved the right side only.

Ear infection, toothache, tension, liver and gall bladder involvement.

This is how localized the zones of disturbance are !

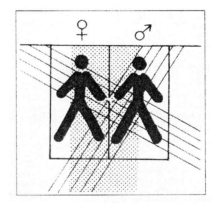

Only on his right side was he exposed to a double influence.

His wife had migraine, depressions, gagging sensations, and anxiety.

After the bed was moved she soon felt better (postcard).

Case# 749. <u>Two crutches and a wheelchair</u>

were needed by Mrs. B. ever since she became 'almost paralysed'.

She reported:

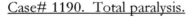

"Eight days after I got married, I started getting ill.

It began with an inflammation of the knee.

After that I had rheumatism. I went through a lot during those 29 years."

"My husband, too, was sick a great deal, his heart and lungs, and he died at an early age.

Our daughter is now sleeping in his bed, and she already has rheumatism."

I recommended that the bed be moved immediately.

Letter: *"All of us feel better now."*

Case# 1190. <u>Total paralysis.</u>

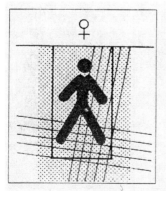

Frau N. (Innsbruck) had been very ill while sleeping in this bed, and during the past 4 years she had been totally paralyzed.

After her mother's death, the daughter began to use the same bed, and she too became ill with abdominal myoma.

She had surgery in 1973.

The bed was moved, and I received a phone call:

"Even the first night I began to sleep better and I feel so much warmer and more comfortable in bed."

Statistical Summary of Cases to No. 1500

B. Geopathic effects on 29 people with eye diseases,

swollen eyelids in the morning, inflammations, nervous blinking, difficulty in focusing when waking up, detached retina (5), blindness (3).

C. Geopathic effects on 123 people with ear, nose, and throat problems.

The following people gave me exact information:

57 :   people with chronic or acute tonsillitis,
         accompanied by high fever
10 :   Tonsillectomy
 4:    Abscessed tonsils
 6:    Chronic hoarseness.
 3:    Feeling of gagging.
 2:    Cancer of the larynx.
16:    Chronic colds.
 3:    Nosebleed so severe as to constitute a threat to life.
 1:    Operation on the nose.
 1 :   Cancer of the nose.
 9:    Ear problems.
10 :   Otitis
 2:    Ringing in the ear.
 8:    Swollen glands
 2:    Tumours.

D. Geopathic effects on 41 persons with teeth, mouth and jaw problems, like inflammations, abscessed teeth or jaws, cysts, neuralgia, cancer of the tongue (2), and grinding of teeth.

E. Geopathic effects on 14 people with skin diseases such as shingles, eczema, psoriasis, skin cancer (5).

F. Geopathic effects on 8 people with bone diseases, bone TB, cancer of the bone (2), osteomyelitis, in 33 people with neck, shoulder, and back pains, in 23 people with disc and spine problems, and in 113 people with lower back problems.

So far I have been able to point to geopathic influences in all cases (12) in which wounds or fractures did not heal for months and sometimes years.

G. Geopathic effects on 76 people with bronchial and lung diseases, like chronic inflammations, TB (20), embolism (2), lung cancer and goitres.

H. Geopathic effects leading to internal disorders:

18 people with thyroid problems
(hyper and hypo functioning).

29 people with asthma.

171 people with heart and circulatory diseases,
such as weakness, palpitations in bed, cramps, tightness
in the chest, inflammations, and infarct (30 cases).

52 people with blood disorders, blood pressure consistently
too high or too low, anaemia, and leukaemia (6).

84 persons with chest diseases, including cancer (20).

84 people with stomach disorders: lack of appetite, nausea,
vomiting, inflammation, tumours (6) , and cancer (10).

67 people with diseases of the colon, such as inflammation,
tumours (6), and other growths, appendicitis (12), chronic
constipation (16), intestinal parasites, intestinal blockage
(5), cancer of the colon (9).

22 people with disorders of the pancreas, such as
inflammation, cancer (5), diabetes (11)

58 people with gall bladder problems, such as inflammation,
vomiting of bile, gallstones, and colic

45 people with liver ailments, such as swollen liver, liver
damage, and cancer of the liver (10).

24 people who are constantly cold in bed.

8 people with profuse perspiration in bed.

5 children with arrested development.

8 people with sudden loss of weight
(up to 20 kilos in 4 weeks).

I. Urology: Geopathic effects in:

67 people with kidney ailments, such as inflammation,
bleeding, formation of pus, kidney stones colics,
and cancer (4).

36 people with bladder problems, like bedwetting (24),
cystitis, stones, and cancer (1).

11 people with prostate problems (3 of them with cancer).

53 people with stomach problems and intestinal problems
without an exact diagnosis.

J. Gynaecology: Geopathic effects on 63 people with abdominal complaints. 6 ovarian problems (cancer in 1).

57   diseases of the uterus, including
3   with polyps,
1   with cysts,
6   with myomas,
8   with cancer, and severe dysmennorhea.

So far it was possible to find detrimental influences from the earth in all cases of spontaneous abortion (14), premature delivery (1), and stillbirth (2).

Four babies died a few days after birth.

The master of dowsing, Adolf Flachenegger, had a list of 47 children whose mothers could conceive and deliver only after years of waiting and only after they had left the area of geopathic influence.

K. Geopathic influence on 180 people with rheumatic diseases, also paralysis.

Five people had total paralysis for many years.

Of those people, two had their beds standing over a 'water crossing' and 3 of them over both a Curry crossing and an underground watercourse (WxCxC).

Summary

In all of the illnesses from A through K, we could ascertain the presence of negative influences from the earth, without a single exception.

Geopathic influences have to be considered among the contributing factors; in 'healthy' people we found negative forces from the earth only rarely (above 50%).

Those people had a great deal of resistance, or had some other external factors working in their favour, like clean mountain air. One might say that they have 'not yet become ill'.

The rule was that the healthy people slept in a 'good' place - my sample of healthy people comprised several thousand cases.

5. Case Studies Concerning Pathogenic Locations
for Sitting and Standing

Locations other than sleeping places, especially working places where people spend several hours a day, can also have a geopathic influence and contribute to ill health.

That will be the case when those places are located over zones of disturbance, and especially over the crossing of these zones of disturbance.

In 37 cases where fainting took place we observed that they all occurred directly above a zone of disturbance.

Usually, however, we also found that those people's resistance was already weakened by nightly influences from pathogenic locations.

After examining more than 500 work places, we can make the following general observations:

People whose permanent place of work is located above a zone of disturbance usually feel uncomfortable, and gradually the amount and speed of work diminish, as well as the quality of the work.

Those people whose permanent place of work is located above a 'radiation-free' area report well-being and they also tend to accomplish tasks faster, have a greater capacity for work, and a higher quality of work.

This is true for all people, but especially, of course, for those who tend to be especially sensitive, or for those who already have health problems.

We have found this to be true for people who work with their hands, as well as for those who work with their intellect.

The latter, provided with a space free of negative radiation, can work at peak performance.

Case# 1084. Fainting spell at the telephone

above a crossing of two water courses and a Curry band.

Three people suffered from fainting spells in Steinach/Brenner:

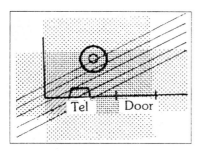

The father died instantaneously. The mother and son were carried away and regained consciousness.

The three incidents happened at different times.

Case# 1486c. A chemist from Salzburg

felt discomfort, registered slight fevers, and was nervous while working at his bench in his laboratory. - many of his experiments failed and had to be repeated.

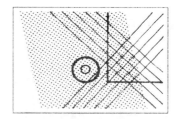

Whenever he worked at a place free of radiation, his experiments proved to be successful.

Case# 759. A banker had occupied a new office for two months.

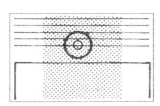

During that time he was unable to work for more than two hours at his desk.

He always got severe pain at the back of his head.

He immediately changed his office and had no more pain from that day on.

Case# 1123. The workplace of a librarian in Austria:

Every evening the librarian felt a slight trembling all over her body and she was extremely tired.

She became very sick.

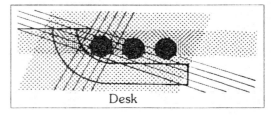

Desk

The library was remodeled, and after that the state of health of the librarian improved greatly.

Case# 899. <u>The operating table in a hospital</u> needs to be located so that it is free of 'radiation'.

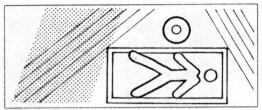

This is of utmost importance for the surgeon, but also for the patient, so that breathing and circulation are in no way impeded.

Case# 1143. <u>In booth No.2 at the post office in Karnten,</u>

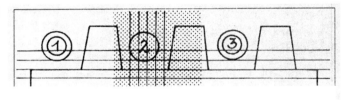

we found that the tellers felt restless, suffered from undefined pains, and took sick leave often.

At booth No.1, they felt well.

Recommendation: Leave booth No.2 free and move to the unoccupied booth No.3.

Case# 1440. <u>Participants at a conference in Brixen/Tyrol</u>

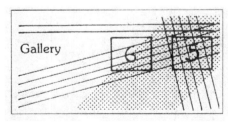

did not feel well in the big conference room.

On seat No.5 the physician felt the place was so 'draughty' that he could not stand it, and he left the room in the middle of a lecture.

Seat No.6: The reporter suffered from headaches the whole day long. Both of those participants felt fine in other places.

Again: very sensitive people, or those with some illness, will register 'not feeling well' even after a short time, if they are located above a zone of water or curry crossings.

Further statistics, their evaluation, and their description are the subject of a later publication.

Only for cancer have we included such an evaluation in Part IV of this book.

Since I am a 'non-medical' scientist, I am not in a position to do valid research into the reason why some patients recover only slowly and partially after their work place has been changed.

Some of them might have suffered permanent damage from the over-use of drugs and other medications.

Part IV - CONCLUSIONS

1. Preventive measures and help through dowsing

The field of neurology can be assisted in the cases of patients who, despite medical treatment, continue to suffer from chronic tension, chronic pain, and certain kinds of depression and apathy.

The simple changing of the position of the bed or the place of work can create the conditions for effective treatment.

Those suffering from migraine headaches are no longer confined to the use of pain relievers, which have serious side effects if taken over a long period of time.

Pediatricians now have a recourse for those children who cry a great deal, sleep restlessly, and get up all the time or run out of their room at night.

It is most important that young children be allowed to live in an atmosphere of peace and safety, without exposure to unknown influences which drain their energies.

Surgery can help patients, especially those who have suffered from cancer, and the process of healing will be accelerated if the attending physician pays attention to the location of the place of rest, in consultation with a dowser.

In the field of internal medicine as well as all the other specialties, physicians have the opportunity to consult an experienced dowser in all cases of uncertain diagnosis or unsatisfactory recovery.

A conscientious physician is not just concerned in treating the symptoms, like fever or swellings, but he searches for the underlying causes and attempts to eliminate them.

Indeed, dowsing does not just offer a valuable tool for the treatment of illnesses, but also for the prevention of illness.

Gynecology can profit in so many cases, heretofore untreatable, by simply ascertaining the need to move the patient's bed to another place in the room or the house.

Damage to the foetus, abortion, prematurity, and prolonged and difficult labour can be prevented in many cases.

It was depressing to listen to the radio on February 22, 1974, to Dr. Rett and Dr. Rosenkrans, who spoke about the damage which premature infants are apt to suffer.

How much dowsing could do for those babies !

I would be happy to send to any interested physician or scientist additional case histories which would fall into their own field of interest.

Or I could send them case histories from any field in which they are interested.

2. Economic Benefits

The Austrian radio news on November 28, 1974, pointed out that rheumatic illnesses are the number one cause for absenteeism from work and that this problem costs the taxpayer millions of dollars per year.

Thus, to pay attention to what dowsing can do would be an advantage not only for the health and well being of people but also for the economy as a whole.

3. The Cancer Problem

I would like to address this problem in particular because of its great importance.

Cancer, even in children comprises the greatest cause of death in Austria, second only to circulatory diseases.

(a). Gustav Baron von Pohl examined, in an official capacity, the Bavarian city of Vilsbiburg with regard to subterranean water currents.

He noted them in the official city map made in 1930.

The health department recorded at the same time, but independently, all those 54 persons who had died of cancer within the past several years, and they noted the living locations of those persons on another map of the city.

There was a surprising agreement in regard to water currents and death from cancer. Those facts were recorded in a protocol.

We have Erica Herbst (Progress for Everyone Publishers, Feucht) to thank for bringing this valuable book to the attention of the public in a new edition 'Earth Rays as Pathogenic Agents in Illness and in Cancer'.

When I did my research work I had no access to this book, and only shortly before the third edition of my book did I have a chance to read about the work of Pohl.

This too pointed to the fact that different dowsers arrive at the same conclusion, independently of one another.

(b). The well-known oncologist Dr. Von Brehmer voiced the opinion in 1932 that the pendulum and the dowsing rod needed to be taken seriously.

(c). Physicians have the following opinions:

Arnold Mannlicher, M.D., wrote in a Swiss medical journal that in 30 years as a practicing physician, **he had not yet found one case of cancer, where there was an absence of influences from the earth.**

He is convinced that cancer is a disease of location and that the influence from the earth has to be considered a substantial factor.

However, other factors must not be underestimated, such as smoking in lung cancer, or strong chemical agents.

Manfred Curry, M.D., wrote in his article (mentioned before) that after a cancer operation, patients have to sleep on a location that is free of disturbances from the earth. He also recommends a special diet for cancer patients.

Josef Issels, M.D., a well-known oncologist, wrote a book meant for physicians and laymen on the subject 'More Cures After Cancer' (Helfer Publishers, Bad Homburg), and devoted a special chapter to the influence of the earth rays: 'The Importance of the Bio-spheres for the Development of Cancer'.

He considers the crossing of the terrestrial rays an important factor in the development of cancer and he sets out to prove this to be so.

He recommends that his chronically sick patients change the place where they sleep and work, to places where the detrimental emanations are absent.

I had the opportunity to meet Dr. Issels personally and after he told me how much he liked my work, he asked me to evaluate his own home.

Dr. Issels pointed out that the well-known surgeons, Dr. Hochenegg and Dr. Nothnagel in Vienna and Dr. Sauerbruch in Berlin, always made sure that the patient would not return to the bed he had slept in previous to the surgery.

They felt that there was hardly any point in doing the surgery unless this important influence was eliminated.

Dr. Dieter Aschoff, M.D. (Wuppertal) wrote an article entitled: 'What are the Questions in Regard to Cancer and the Zones of Disturbance ?' in which he reported:

"Despite decades of painstaking oncological research, science has not yet been able to find a cause for cancer, with the exception of cancer through ionising radiation, such as X rays, radium emissions, or other kinds of cancer caused by rays.

Yet the cases of cancer which can be attributed to those causes are actually very small, and science is still confronted with the unsolved cause of cancer.

But earth rays are ionising rays also, and they have to be recognized in scientific circles as causes of cancer."

At a lecture in Dortmund, May 15, 1976, Dr. Aschoff reported that he himself had measured with a UKW instrument the bed sites of 30 patients, and **he had not seen one case of a chronically ill patient where there was not a measurable zone involved.**

He reported further: *"In 1934 Dr. Rambeau, president of the Marburg medical society, published the results of his measurements which he conducted with instruments, and **concluded that all of the cancer cases he investigated had slept above measurable zones of disturbance.***

In those houses where there were no such influences, the people enjoyed good health."

In 1939 Cody presented the results of his seven years of research in Le Havre.

In over 10,000 measurements above the beds of oncological patients he found vertical ionizing rays which reach the upper floors and can easily be detected with instruments.

Ionizing rays are the only cause for cancer which so far have been recognized the world over.

Dieter Aschoff, M.D., has also been the first person to make use of the electromagnetic oscillations of the blood, which are physically measurable, in the blood drop test.

People with electrically oscillating blood were found to live without exception over geopathic zones of disturbance, either where they slept, or where they worked.

And those people whose blood was magnetically oscillating were not exposed to geopathic disturbances and were free of illness.

Dr. Aschoff - and now also other physicians, including Dr. Morrell, Dr. Rossaint, Dr. Rotdach in Munich, Dr. Alfred Lautner in Vienna (these names do not exhaust the list of those who have availed themselves of these tests) - have done remarkable work by using the blood drop test for the early recognition of illnesses and also for the appropriate choice of medication.

Thus, this method lends itself particularly well to the early recognition of cancer and thus can mean a chance of recovery from cancer.

Dr. Aschoff advises that to learn how to administer the blood drop test is not difficult for a physician, but that an introductory course is mandatory.

I personally would recommend all interested physicians, physicists, dowsers, and laypeople to study the lectures given by Dr. Aschoff on the subject, and in particular the lectures 'Electromagnetic Properties of the Blood Become Measurably Altered Through the Influences of Zones of Disturbance' and 'The Electromagnetic Blood Test'.

Dr. Hartmann in Eberbach examined the sleeping places of his cancer patients with the ultra high frequency field detector.

He writes: "It was very disturbing that among the many sleeping places occupied by cancer patients, there was not a single one which did not register a strong reaction exactly at the site of the cancer.

The cancer problem is a geopathic stress problem and therefore a preventative environmental issue.

The German naturopath Hans Schumann (Lauf/Pegnitz) wrote in his book 'Successful Treatment of Cancer Through Biological Methods Involving the Whole Person' (Veritas Verlag, Linz,) that in his practice he saw that in all cases of cancer geopathic influences had to be considered to be partially responsible for the illness.

As soon as his patients changed the place where they slept, there were always remarkable improvements made in the way they felt.

I recommend Hans Schumann's book very highly, since it describes the utilization of natural healing agents, based on scientific research, and it includes special diets as well as the necessity for psychological support.

This book is understandable for the layman and has many pictures to aid its comprehensiveness.

Of course, cancer patients must remain with their physician or the person who previously took care of them medically.

(d). All the 'biological dowsers' like Abbe Mermet (Switzerland), Adolf Flachenegger, Hugo Wurm (Linz), Johanna Langsenlehner (Austria), Dr. Czepl and Richard Meisinger (Vienna), the late Joseph Rehr (Salzburg - *I think of him with much gratitude, since he saved me from the influence of the zones of disturbance many years ago*), and the many German dowsers, among them Bernhard Peters, who sent my book all over the world, and so many others - **all of them have observed after critical examination of so many apartments and houses of cancer patients and those who died of cancer, that there is always a geopathic zone of disturbance present.**

I myself was able to ascertain this fact in 500 cases of cancer and other cell growths.

I have never found a case where geopathic zones of disturbance were not present.

Yes, even when we observed certain 'cancer places' where several people, one after the other, contracted cancer, or where several people became ill on different floors of the same building while sleeping at the same spot one beneath the other.

These are not hypotheses, but facts !

A letter of Prof. Alois Felder, M.D. (Linz):

"I just put down your book again. The wife of my nephew just told me in tears that her twin brother had suddenly died and that he had suffered from severe headaches.

He was only 25 years old.

While living in his old home, he was always a healthy and energetic person.

But when he moved into a new house in 1975 he developed strange symptoms for which no cause could be found.

During the autopsy a tumour was found which had caused this quick and agonizing death.

I asked to be shown the room in which he had slept.

I picked up my dowsing rod.

The room was so intensely 'disturbed' that the rod reacted violently about every half metre, especially where his head used to be.

After ten minutes of work in this room, I was so totally exhausted and trembling that I had to give up any further investigations of it.

This particular result and so many others which I cannot even enumerate here constitute such an obligation for me to do still more in this field. I am asking for your assistance."

Again, so that there is no misunderstanding, I want to reiterate:

We do not claim that every zone of disturbance will result in cancer - rather, we have found zones of disturbance in every case of cancer.

We are well aware that there are other factors that come into play in the development of cancer.

But at the same time, it is of such importance to consider the contribution which the crossings of zones of disturbance make in the formation of cancer, that science can no longer afford to ignore those influences !

I was very upset when I realized at the Oncology Conference (1979, Baden-Baden) how powerless medicine still is in regard to cancer.

I assume it has to do with not searching for the root, the cause of the illness.

At the same time, I have to consider the fact that I was invited to this congress and was even asked to contribute to the discussion by showing slides about my cancer case histories and their connection with crossings of zones of disturbance.

That fact alone shows me that the leading scientists and physicians are becoming more willing to consider dowsing and other methods not strictly connected with traditional medical practice.

It is important that our contribution leads to a different attitude toward the phenomenon of cancer.

Again, I want to emphasize that, of course, to bring about cure in any illness, and especially in cancer, it is not enough to move the bed in order to get well.

Rather, a rigorous and conscientious medical regime must be adhered to as well.

It is just our observation that medical treatment can become effective, once the disturbing influence of geopathy is removed.

At the same time, nowadays more than ever before, it would behoove everyone to lead a healthful life and to become a collaborator in their own health.

Health insurance companies would welcome such an attitude too !

I want to cite a few books which I consider sound and important.

'Cancer, Leukaemia: Suggestions for Prophylaxis and Treatment_of Many Illnesses'. Rudolf Breuss, Walter Margreiter

'Helping and Healing'. P. Thomas Haberle. Veritas Publishers

'More Cancer Cures'. Joseph Issels, M.D. Heifer Publishing

'Checkmate Cancer'. Dr. Kuhl. Humata Publishers

'Good Health from Nature'. Hans Neuner. Perlinger Publishers

'Successful Treatment of Cancer Through Biological-Holistic Treatments'. Hans Schumann. Healthy Living Publishers

'Health Through God's Pharmacy'. Maria Treben. Ennsthaler

(e). Two German universities, the Public Health Institute in Heidelberg, and an Institute at the University for Technology in Munich, studied plants and animals in regard to disturbing influences from the earth and confirmed the previous findings: 'Cancer is definitely linked to geopathic influences'

(f). Modern cancer research has finally recognized the necessity of getting the body to mobilize its own resistance.

This was the topic of discussion during the Oncology meeting in 1973 in Baden-Baden. Israeli cancer researchers made the same statement (April 24, 1974).

Normally, the body will recognize foreign cells and will destroy them.

But the body which is already sick, is unable to recognize them and so destroy them.

Thus the cancer cells continue to multiply and to grow.

It is of great importance to help the cancer patient to a greater degree of resistance.

In a radio interview, I heard a university professor from Graz lament that apathy was one of the greatest evils of our time, in important aspects as well as in minor ones, and that so many excuses turn out to be simple matters of convenience.

That same apathy he blames also for the inability to recognize cancer in its earliest stages.

There is a growing consensus that the development of cancer is dependent essentially on the degree of immunity of the body.

Now that this fact is becoming more and more recognized, we can hope that the next step will follow soon: namely, the avoidance of negative influences from the earth so that the body can achieve the desired resistance.

(g). Statistics.

Cancer and other Cell Growths (carcinoma, myomas, polyps, tumours)

The first 150 people I investigated with neoplasms were exposed to the following influences:

W	0
C	0
WxC	39
CxC	13
WxW	12
WxCxC	69
WxWxC	10
WxWxCxC	7
Total:	150

All the cases exhibiting cell growth (including cancer) were located directly above a zone of disturbance (100%).

Those 150 cases were statistically evaluated.   An additional 350 cases of cell growth confirm the same experience.

I want to emphasize again that, of course, other factors also play an important part in the development of cell growths.

4. Suggestions

I am always asked to make some practical suggestions; these are the primary ones.

(a). It would be of great importance to disseminate this information and thus influence public opinion, and to make contact with traditional practitioners of medicine so that universities and teachers of medical schools could incorporate this information into their curriculum.

It is important to support financially the research done in the field of dowsing with research grants, workshops for the dowsers, and the hiring of dowsers by the public.

They could show adequate training by working towards a recognized degree.

(b). Disseminate this knowledge by telling other people about it.

People should not only feel free, but should rather feel compelled, to inform their friends and acquaintances in regard to geopathic influences, and thus help many people who are sick and suffering.

We should all defend those people who are branded as hypochondriacal, hysterical, or malingering.

We should be willing to point out that there might be a geopathic factor affecting them.

Pastoral counsellors, too, might incorporate into their work the possibility of zones of disturbance in cases of depression and suicidal tendencies.

They might recommend moving the bed to another location.

I want to draw attention to Pfarrer Kneipp, who was as concerned about the physical well-being of his patients as he was about their spiritual well-being.

He recognized the healing powers of water and used them, while the dowser's task is to point out the destructive force inherent in water.

Physicians ought to consider geopathic influences as one possible cause of illness, and should recommend moving of the bed on a trial basis.

In general, people should trust their own powers of observation more.

Dowsers and physicians should always encourage people to notice incidents in their own families and among their friends and acquaintances, such as whether there might be sleeping or working places where several people in succession have suffered from severe illness and consequent death.

In order to avoid further catastrophes, these people need to be urged to move the bed at least one to two metres.

Teachers could give short presentations at various conferences about geobiological influences, and high school students should have this knowledge available in their biology curriculum.

A colleague of mine came up with this idea and did just that, using this book as required reading.

5. Promising Prospects

(a). 'Moving the bed just in case' is helpful.

I want to emphasize this fact, especially for those people who are chronically ill.

The probability is very high that they will experience relief when the bed, or the place of work, is moved, often only one or two metres.

It will depend on where they experience their discomfort.

That is enough, in most cases.

Only then can a medical treatment become successful.

I know of many such cases, where the physician gave such advice and thus was able finally to achieve a cure, or at least a real improvement.

I have given the same advice in lectures and in letters.

I have plenty of written proof in my possession.

Some of those I have already mentioned, but I want to quote five more:

A university professor (Karnten) who suffered from severe sleep disturbance wrote:

"Ever since I moved my bed, just in case, I have been able to sleep very well."

A young woman wrote that she had given the same advice to a friend, a woman who was constantly sick and who never felt well, and that this friend was feeling very much better.

I have two cases of mothers who read the advice in a popular magazine and who then moved the beds of their sons and enjoyed remarkable success.

One mother, the wife of a university professor, wrote to me that she moved her 10 year old son's bed back to the old place, since he had suffered from insomnia and school failures for the past few years.

She was able to see that his headaches subsided, that he slept better, and that he did well in his oral exams which took place soon after the bed was moved.

The other mother, after a lecture in Mondsee shared with the audience that she, too, upon reading the report in the magazine, moved the bed of her cranky and unhappy five year old.

He now sleeps through the night and is doing much better in general.

I want to thank the journalist Gunther Winklbauer for his article in the 'Bunten Illustrierten' entitled 'Blame the Desk for Your Poor Grade' (Oct. 18, 1973).

The responses to his courageous declaration, which were sent to me, proved that his efforts had fallen on fertile ground.

As the fifth case I want to mention the written confirmation of a kindergarten teacher:

"I suffered for years from the most terrible nightmares.

I was really quite desperate. I heard that one cause might be some detrimental influence from the earth, and since I did not have anything to lose, I moved my bed.

Ever since then I have slept well and have had no nightmares at all!"

I am sure that this teacher will tell the mother and fathers of her pupils about geopathic influences and what results a simple measure like moving the bed can bring.

I am delighted about every case I am told about where a 'moving of the bed for good measure' resulted in improvement.

(b). The 'location test' is often successful.

Many people are able to look for and find a 'good place' for themselves.

All that is needed is patience, goodwill, and a few hours of undisturbed time.

Sensitive people and those with ill-defined pains are very good candidates for this test.

Standing quietly, or sitting on a wooden chair, one examines the whole bedroom slowly, while listening to one's body, in a relaxed and carefree manner (not anxious and tense), moving a few feet at a time and taking notes.

Wherever one feels well one can remain for ten minutes or so.

But at those places where one cannot breathe well, where one does not feel well, where one gets tingling sensations, pulling, cramps, pains in the region of the heart, or other pains, one needs to leave right away.

One needs only about two square metres for the bed (6 x 3 ft), and the chances are that one can find a healthful location.

Thus everyone can help himself, even without the aid of a dowser.

The dowser should be called only in particularly difficult cases when a 'location test' does not bring the desired results.

Again, many notes and letters attest to the fact that adults as well as children are able to find for themselves their 'good' sleeping place with the aid of this test, and that their health improves and many students show improved grades and test scores.

For several years now I have invited the occupants of an apartment, after I have done the examination, to close their eyes and to feel the good places.

Almost everyone is able to accomplish this test satisfactorily.

At first they tend to be skeptical, and also surprised, and then they become enthusiastic about their discovery and exclaim:

"Well, now we are perfectly willing to put in the effort connected with moving the bed to another place."

The dowser can consider the results the people reach by feeling the place as a proof of his own investigation.

(c). Minor disturbances are easy to tolerate for all of us.

Most people are not exposed to the crossings of different zones of disturbance, but rather to minor influences.

While going through my cases one could gain the erroneous impression that the majority of mankind is exposed to such 'crossings' since I cited all those examples.

That is definitely not correct.

But to strengthen my argument and to convince the scientists, it was necessary to illustrate my point with so many extreme case histories.

Most people do not need to sleep or to work at a place completely free of radiation.

Minor influences from zones of disturbance are tolerable in most cases, especially when it is recognized that a healthful and peaceful life-style will counteract whatever damage might ensue from earth radiations.

This is an observation which I have made in very many cases.

Not only the professional associations of dowsers, but many other associations and organizations will provide their members with lectures, courses, and magazines on means for a healthier way of life.

For those interested readers, I have listed the names and addresses of those associations with which I am familiar. [Not included in this edition]

As far as I know their reading material can also be ordered by non-members.

Finally I would like to emphasize that I have in no way exhausted all the damaging environmental influences, or all the other influences to which we humans are subjected.

I have only been concerned with showing the geopathic influence of the water currents and the curry net.

The day will come when the influences from the earth cannot be denied any longer, but will get full attention.

At the same time, those in responsible positions will be willing to make use of the contribution which well-planned dowsing can make.

Electromagnetic waves have been in existence for billions of years, but only in our century have their importance and usefulness been recognized (radio, television, telephone).

The existence of influences from the earth has been known to different people for thousands of years.

Perhaps it is up to our century to explore and understand these forces and to become cognizant of their influence on people.

I hope that my work is a building block toward this end.

Please don't put this book down feeling anxious that there are zones of disturbance, but rather full of joy and gratitude that we and those who suffer from illness and depression can so easily find good places in which to live.

If we follow, despite all the damage which is being done to the environment, the advice of the geobiologists, environmentalists, and health-conscious architects and designers, and if we give credence to our innate sensitivities, then we and those around us with thankfulness toward God, will be able to experience once again:

Peace and Salvation.

ABOU BEN ADAM - Son of Adam

Abou ben Adam, may his tribe increase
Awoke one night from a dream of peace
And saw in the moonlight of his room -
Making it rich, like a lily in bloom -
An Angel writing in a book of gold.
Exceeding peace made Ben Adam bold
To the presence in the room he said
"What writest thou ?" - The Angel raised his head
And replied, with a look of sweet accord,
"The names of those who Love the Lord".
"And is mine one ?" spoke Abou. "Nay, not so"
Replied the vision. Abou spoke more low,
But cheerily still, and said: "I pray thee, then,
Write me as one who loves his fellow men"
The Angel wrote and vanished. The next night
It came again with a great waking Light
And showed the names whom Love of God had Blessed.
Lo ! Ben Adam's name led all the rest.

Further Thoughts

By John Living, Professional Engineer

The Book

This book is, without any doubt, the classic record of the effect of noxious earth energies upon human health; it is a faithful record of illnesses found due to people spending a lot of their time in a place where they are subjected to 'Earth Radiations' that are noxious to them.

The book was written in German by Käthe Bachler in 1976, translated into English by Marianne Gerhart in 1984, and published in English by Wordmasters in 1989.

This edition is being published some 30 years after the original German version, thanks to the kindness of the holders of the copyrights to the earlier English version - which has long been out of print; second hand copies have been sold on ebay for US$89 !

The latest statistics show that the death rates related to cancer in North America have grown from the previous estimate of 25% to a new high in 2007 of 33%.

Reports are that when gypsies in Europe were surveyed, less than 2% had a family member who suffered from cancer; perhaps this is due to them being more 'aware' of these noxious earth energies, and to their constant movement from place to place.

Noxious Earth Energies

Note that I am using the term 'noxious earth energies' instead of 'earth radiation'. To me, the term 'radiation' involves rays that radiate in all directions, similar to the rays of light given by a light bulb.

The term currently used in most English speaking countries is 'Noxious Earth Energies'. 'Noxious' meaning detrimental to your health and well-being.

The noxious earth energies seem to operate in vertical bands, and not radiate outside such bands; they affect residents of a penthouse in a high-rise apartment just as much as those who live in the basement suite.

The Curry Grid seems to be running NW-SE and NE-SW, diagonally to the North, East, South, and West directions; the energy bands are not very wide, and seem to be running about 3 metres - 10 feet apart.

The lines also alternate in character; in esoteric terms, a Yang (positive) grid line adjoins a Yin (negative) grid line, running in opposite directions, i.e. from NW to SE, then from SE to NW.

Where these lines cross, or interact with the energy bands from noxious water, an energy vortex seems to be formed - similar to the vortex of a tornado, but on a smaller scale.

Since these grid lines are so close together, it would be expected that every person would be affected - and this would be so if all the grid lines were equally noxious. So why are not all persons made ill ?

It seems that the grid system is similar to that of roads in a city - you have residential roads, collector roads, and highways. For the Curry Grid, there may be a collector road for every so many residential road, and a highway for every so many collector roads.

The degree of noxiousness in a Curry Grid line is similar to the amount of traffic carried by such roads - and if you sleep in the middle of a highway, you are sure to get run over !

Hence it is needed not only to identify if a Curry Line exists where time is spent, but also to quantify its strength - and hence its likely effect, its degree of noxiousness.

Water veins may be just a tiny trickle running way below the surface; it seems that the quantity of flow and its depth have little bearing on the noxious strength.

The essential need is to identify if any noxious energies are located where a person is sleeping or sitting for a long time, determine the noxious strength, locate the positions of these energies, and to take appropriate action.

Because this is so important (and relatively easy for all of us to do) a section explaining how you can do most of this yourself is included.

This includes learning to Dowse, and how you can use this skill, abstracted from my book 'Intuition Technology' - which explains how you can use Dowsing in many more ways, including Healing.

Human Bodies

Unless a person is stuck in a refusal to accept evidence, it must be acknowledged that our bodies are made of energy, and surrounded by other energy bodies not normally perceived by normal sight.

These auric bodies have been described by many people who have the ability to see them, and have been 'captured' by Kirlian photography.

Our bodies also have energy systems that are not in the physical plane, such as meridians and Chakras; we cannot see them, or find them when a body is dissected - but we cannot see X-rays or radio waves either. But we accept that they exist.

It may well be that the strong energy vortexes that are formed at the noxious energy junctions interfere with the energy patterns of our bodies - and hence cause disruptions in our systems, leading to illness.

I am reminded of one case reported on the internet: parents took a healthy baby on a visit, and parked the pram in the shade of a tree which was badly mis-shapen. Half an hour later, they found their baby dead.

It was ascertained that the tree had been twisted by noxious earth energies, and that these were so strong that the baby could not survive even such a short time in their field.

One wonders how many cases of 'Sudden Infant Death' are also attributable to exposure to noxious earth energies.

We All are Intuitive !

Have you ever felt 'that something is wrong !', walked into a room and felt a 'bad atmosphere', met a person for the first time and felt your body sway towards them (attraction) or away (repulsion - their energy is not compatible with yours) ? If so, this demonstrates that you have worked with your Intuition.

We all have the simple physical senses: sight, hearing, feeling, taste, smell, and balance (yes - balance is our sixth sense !), but teachers and lecturers know that to 'get a point across' they have to appeal to the prominent senses of the audience - some people have a very strong visual sense, or need to 'feel' the subject matter.

It seems that we all have Souls (or more correctly, are Souls having an experience in a human body) and that our Soul has its own set of senses.

When the subject matter is presented in the way that responds best to the dominant 'Soul Sense' then the message does 'get across'.

Our Intuition may well be from a 'Higher Level Being', such as a guide or Guardian Angel, trying to help us - if we listen, or are otherwise aware of the communication. Our Intuition is 'above' our senses, and uses these in various ways to communicate.

It seems that our Heart is our major link to our Intuition; when we use our logical Mind-Brain team to form a question and then ask the question to our Heart (just by imagining that we are 'talking' to our Heart) then our Heart-Mind-Brain team uses our nervous-muscular system to signal a response.

This usually starts with a body movement forwards for YES or backwards for NO. But we can define other signals, such as the number of eye blinks or the movement of our tongue, to give the signal - so long as we have specified the signal to be used and its meaning to our Heart-Mind-Brain team.

The question must be clear and precise, without any double meanings, and is best formed in simple language such as a four or five year old child would understand, to yield a YES or a NO answer. We should concentrate our thought on the question.

By thinking of a particular person or effect we are 'tuning' our Heart-Mind-Brain team to the specific vibrational pattern which identifies the subject of our thought - like tuning a radio to a station.

The context of the question (and answer) must be within your understanding; if your are asking about a health problem or sub-atomic physics, then you should have knowledge and experience in that field - and will be able to ask questions of greater depth.

For asking a more complicated question, the game of 'Twenty Questions' (or Animal, Vegetable, Mineral) can be used. When an answer is received, be aware of any 'very first thought' that 'pops' into your head - it is probably a 'hint' from your Intuition.

This is a very quick summary - for a more detailed explanation see my book: Intuition 'On Demand'. This includes advice as to 'questions not to ask', programming your Heart-Mind-Brain team, and simple Dowsing.

When working with our Heart-Mind-Brain team it is important to check: *"Show me the signal for YES"*, then *".. NO"*, *"Was the answer correct ?"*, and *"Did I understand the answer correctly ?"*.

Experimenting with Other Noxious Energies

It is not only some earth energies that are noxious to humans - electro-magnetic radiation from Cathode Ray Tube television and computer screens can cause problems.

When we have knowledge of these and tune our minds to these energies, we can feel them with our hands.

As an experiment, keep a thought of these electro-magnetic energy emissions and approach the area in front of a switched-on CRT screen from the side, holding one of your hands in front of you with its palm facing forwards.

Can you feel any slight difference as you move forward ?

You may find that the air seems slightly more dense (or resistant to your movement) as you move towards the area right in front of the screen.

If you repeat this at a distance further from the TV, the effect can still be felt, but not as strongly.

If you can feel this energy with your hands, be sure that the organs within your body that find this energy to be detrimental will be even more sensitive to the energy.

One way to check if your bed or chair is in a zone of noxious energy is to use this procedure, keeping a thought of 'noxious energy' in your Heart-Mind-Brain team, and feel for any changes 'in the air' around your bed or chair.

You do not have to be an expert of noxious energy to do this - your body is very aware of any noxious effect !

Another way is to stand at the foot of your bed, or in front of your chair (home or office), and ask your Heart "Is there any energy zone on any part of my bed (or chair) that is noxious to me ?".

You can also quantify any of these noxious energies, by asking "Is this noxious energy causing serious illness to me ?" remembering that although your body may have reserves to overcome the effect, those reserves are not limitless - so the noxious energy may have a bad effect that worsens as time progresses.

Disease may result quickly in an environment of strong noxious energy, or may manifest over a number of years where they are weaker.

If you usually lie down in a way that avoids a particular area of your bed, or fail to wake up feeling refreshed, take this as a warning that your bed may be in a bad location - and check the position.

These 'drawdowns' of your reserves are cumulative; if you have bad positions for your bed and for any other place where you remain for a considerable time, then the combined drawdown may exceed your ability for replenishment.

If your body sways forward to give a YES signal, then imagine that your bed or chair is in another position, and repeat the question for that location. Imagine different locations until you find one that is free of noxious energy.

Now you may still have a problem - if your partner sleeps with you, s/he may still be in a zone of noxious energy, although you would be free ! So repeat the exercise asking about your partner - hopefully finding a position that is safe for you both.

For your children and your other relations, do this exercise again remembering to substitute their name in the question asked.

In my book, 'Intuition Technology', written as the course manual for teaching Dowsing, I give some proven methods of locating, identifying, and quantifying noxious energies, and ways to work with these energies to reduce or eliminate their noxiousness - without having to move the bed or chair. These are included to help you.

Even X-rays used in dentistry and medical diagnosis have an effect on the energies of a human being. Even in small doses, it seems that the effect includes disruption of communication between the X-rayed cells and the health co-ordinating systems of the body - resulting in the cells exhibiting inappropriate behaviour.

I wonder if one reason for the current increase in breast cancer may be due to the increased X-ray scans being made on women ?

We can help alleviate this sort of problem by telling 'all the life forms within our body' that we love them, and ask that they all 're-establish good communication with our good health system'.

Some exceptional clairvoyants have noted that all cancer affected cells are spiraling anti-clockwise; so it may also help if you ask all your cells to spiral clockwise - the way that all healthy cells are reported to spiral. Our cells have life - they are life forms !

Dowsing (English) / Radiesthesia (Some Other Languages)

Käthe Bachler repeats a belief held many years ago - that only 'sensitive' people are able to Dowse. But we are all sensitive to some degree and in various ways - and can improve our sensitivity.

You have been successful in the experiment to locate noxious energies, so you now know that you have this ability. The system that you used is called 'Deviceless Dowsing' because you are not using any tool or device except your own body.

Some of the best teachers of Dowsing have found that teaching their students to locate noxious energies is the best way to get people started in Dowsing - the human body is so very responsive to these energies !

My experience in teaching Dowsing is that about 90% of people can learn to Dowse; if they cannot learn, it is usually because of some belief that is against Dowsing - and so interferes with their ability.

My name for Dowsing is 'Intuition Technology'. My explanation is that it is using tools to amplify the signals given by our nervous-muscular system as directed by our Heart-Mind Brain team.

Using tools has one extra advantage - that they can be used to point: to indicate a direction, select one of a set of answers, and signal the strength of a force - such as the effect of a noxious energy.

Everything (including atoms and sub-atomic particles) exist because of the vibrational patterns that form them, and have attributes according to the effects of these vibrational patterns or 'Dances of Energy'.

So we can 'tune' our Heart-Mind Brain team to any of these vibrational patterns and communicate with them to some extent, depending upon our 'fine tuning' capability.

Aggression will develop resistance; approaching these 'intelligences' with Love and asking for their help yields positive results. This is important in our own approach to healing within ourselves.

We can use this skill to make lists of things and correctly identify where problems exist - such as deficiencies of vitamins or trace elements, causes of illness, appropriate medicines to be taken - and the doses and frequency needed.

This method is often used in determining the cause of allergies - using kinesiology (muscle testing) which is a form of Dowsing.

Amplifying Intuitive Signals

It is most important to remember that Intuitive signals are originated by our Heart-Mind-Brain team (our Heart being our Intuitive link to 'Upstairs', working closely with the Intuitive part of our Mind-Brain) and then manifested by our nervous-muscular system to give physical movements in our bodies.

In many cases this is done by manipulating the use of our real sixth physical sense - our sense of balance; we have balance sensors throughout our bodies, and these may be used to give a slight twisting of your arm, wrist, and hand muscles.

These signals given by our sense of balance can be amplified by the use of simple tools such as an L-rod or a Pendulum.

Intuition on Building Sites

You will find many plumbers, electrical workers, and water-works employees who use a piece of bent wire - it is cheap, does not break, is easy to carry, simple to use, and proven to be effective.

They use it to locate water pipes and buried wires - they have success even when the original engineering drawings were incorrect or have been lost. Beyond just locating the pipe or wire, they can even locate the spot where there is a leak or break.

This 'Pipe Locator' is usually a length of strong wire (perhaps a welding rod) bent in a 'L' shape - the shorter length being the handle, and the longer length the pointer.

It needs to be held correctly; the operator's elbow should be loose at his side, with the forearm, wrist, and hand extended forward. The handle should hold the handle strongly enough to give good support, but loosely enough so that the pointer can swing easily.

To start, the pointer is guided to be pointing forwards; this means that it is hanging down slightly, so that gravity keeps it forward - but not hanging down so far that it will not sway when the operator's wrist and hand give a slight twist.

The operator tunes his Heart-Mind-Brain 'radio', concentrating his thoughts to whatever is being sought, such as picturing a pipe - or water leaking from a pipe.

Now he walks slowly forward, and the pointer may swing (usually in, towards his body centre) to indicate that his Heart-Mind-Brain has found resonance between the tuned thought and what is being sought; then the operator marks this point on the ground in some way.

It is customary to then approach this point from the opposite side, and locate a similar point of first contact. The item being sought can generally be found half way between these two points of first contact, and a depth equal from either first point of contact to the centre, the half-way point - and this position is also marked.

This whole procedure may be repeated at other places nearby, to confirm the location of the pipe or wire.

If a leak or break is sought, the operator will then follow along the indicated location of the pipe or wire, picturing the leak or break in his Mind, and using his wire (sometimes called an L-rod) as before - to find where it is.

Making your L-Rod

If you do not have an L-rod, get hold of a metal coat hanger, cut off the hook section, and cut the bottom bar in the centre; you now have two pieces of wire - bend then so that they form a right angle at the bend, and you now have two L-rods.

Wire with 90° bend

Half drinking straw as a handle, put the uncut end uppermost, make a bend below to keep it in place.

If you wish, you can cut a drinking straw in two, and slip each half over a handle of your L-rods - keep the uncut edge uppermost - if the cut edge rubs against the pointer it may catch and stop free rotation.

Signals for your L-Rod

The basic signals for use with an L-rod are 'joining is positive, separation is negative'. The amount of movement, the degree of change, indicates the strength of the signal.

If we imagine our L-rod to be the hour hand of a clock, with the 12 o'clock mark furthest from us, then movement between the 11 and 1 marks indicates searching - trying to get the answer, and not the answer itself.

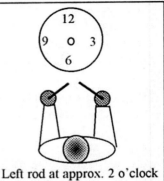

With your L-rod held in your right [left] hand, 10 [2] indicates a weak YES, with the strength rising to a strong YES at 8 [4]. If it goes to 7 [5] this is a 'YES-beyond-YES', a better than expected result. The signals for NO are reversed: 2 - 4 [10 - 8], with 'NO-beyond-NO' at 5 [7].

Left rod at approx. 2 o'clock
Right rod at about 10 o'clock

Many people use an L-rod in each hand; the advantage is that you get confirmation when they both give the same answer. Should they differ, check your question, or stand up and ask your Heart the same question and see whether you move forwards or backwards.

In all such cases, be aware of the very first thought that 'pops' into your Mind - this comes from your Intuition, and will probably assist you to correct any problem with your question.

Is the Baby a Boy ?

There are many stories of ladies holding a needle and thread over a future mother's stomach and asking this question - and they are surprisingly correct most of the time !

If there is an error, it is usually in the question asked - *"Is it a boy or a girl ?"* will give a YES signal, because it could be either.

Sometimes a pendant, crystal on a chain, or other type of Pendulum is used. The item used is not important - it is just a tool being used by the Heart-Mind-Brain team via the nervous-muscular system, again using the balance receptors to cause movements of the forearm, wrist, and hand.

The manipulation of these is far more complicated than with an L-rod, but the principle remains the same.

The signals used may vary; this does not matter, so long as they are understood by the operator. The operator may even decided to change the signals or their meaning - and this works, so long as the sub-conscious Mind understands the new system.

This method is also used in many egg hatcheries to determine the sex of the unborn chicks - again with great success, even on a commercial basis.

The signals are usually based on the subject or answer being Positive/YES or Negative/NO. This Positive/Negative is like comparing the direction of a flow - from the positive to the negative.

Male is generally seen by the Heart-Mind-Brain team as being positive, giving out energy; Female is seen as negative in the sense of being receptive.

A Pendulum is able to move in more directions than an L-rod, so the signaling can be more extensive - swinging to and fro in various directions, or rotating clockwise or anti-clockwise, or even making elliptical combinations of these movements. Again, the strength of the movement indicates the strength of the answer.

Basically, there are two major systems of signaling - these as being the Physical and the Meta-Physical systems.

The Physical system is similar to that used by L-rods - to and fro indicates a joining (the food is good for you to eat), side to side a separation (a barrier between the food and yourself - do not eat it ! - for whatever reason).

The Meta-Physical system is rotational - YES, positive, male, inputting an energy, and sending Love being clockwise; NO, negative, female, extracting an energy being anti-clockwise. Note that there is no 'taking of Love' !

A signaling system that I find excellent is YES = clockwise, NO = anti-clockwise, WAITING = to and fro, NOT AVAILABLE = side to side. These are all simple movements, that cannot be mistaken.

This method of working with your Intuition is generally called 'Radiesthesia', 'Dowsing', or sometimes when locating wells 'Water Witching'.

Signal Training for your Pendulum

You can make a Pendulum by any form of weight suspended by a flexible connector that you can hold in your hand. You can tie a piece of string around a metal nut, for example.

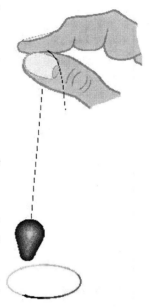

You can also use a crystal on a chain, a cross or other neck decoration, or a glass bead on a length of cord. Some people use specially shaped Pendulums - because energies are very responsive to shapes, to forms of structure.

But even so, the main movement originates from your Heart-Mind-Brain team via your nervous-muscular system - YOU are the most important part!

You will find it best to hold your Pendulum with the string, cord, or chain between your thumb and first finger, as shown.

A long length of string enables you to see the movement more easily, but the speed of movement is slow. A very short length moves very fast, but the amount of movement is less, making it more difficult to see - a real problem when you are starting!

Probably the best length to use when starting is about six inches (15 cm) - then as you get more experienced, you can reduce this to between 3 and 4 inches (7 and 10 cm), as you find suits you.

Some LOLs (Little Old Ladies) are absolute wizards at using a Pendulum; their friends may watch them, and try to do the same: *"It doesn't work for me!"* they cry. Why is this so?

In most cases this is because they have not trained their system to give signals. This is like telling a five year old child *"Give me the first five numbers in the Fibonacci series"* - he does not have any idea of what is meant, which of his toys you want.

Now it may work if you ask your Heart *"Please give me a signal with my Pendulum that indicates YES"* and the watch to see if your Pendulum moves. Repeat the question for NO, and for NOT AVAILABLE, and remember the signals. Then you can ask questions.

It may be best to decide which signal you want to use, and then train your Heart-Mind-Brain team and your nervous-muscular system to give these. I find the following best:

NOT AVAILABLE	Side to side swing
WAITING	To and fro swing
YES	Clockwise circle
NO	Anticlockwise circle

So for each of these signals, make your Pendulum give the signal by using all your muscles in your forearm, wrist, and hand - exaggerating these movements (since you are in a training session) and saying *"This is a [to and fro swing], it signals [WAITING] !"*, and then holding your Pendulum still, and asking *"Please give me the signal for [WAITING]"*.

Repeat this until you get a good response for the signal being installed, and then do the same training session for the next signal, until they are all satisfactory.

It is best to do these in the order shown, since you can go into the WAITING mode before getting the other signals - it is easier for your Pendulum to change its movement rather than start from being still.

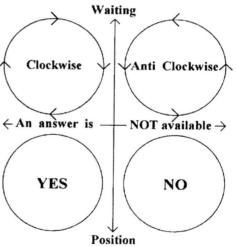

Pointing - with your Pendulum

One of the very good reasons for using a circle to signal YES or NO is that when you seek ask your Pendulum to point towards something you can check that it is giving a good signal.

Define the signal used by your Dowsing system: *"When my Pendulum points to an item, it will first give a YES signal to indicate that it is the correct direction, or a NO signal to show that a problem exists"*.

A linear signal for YES or NO could be confused with the direction sought - the circular signals avoid this problem.

Your Pendulum swings in two directions - if so you are you must then point to one of them with your hand and ask *"Is this the correct direction ?"*

Simple Counting

A simple way of getting experience with pointing is to practice with this 'Counting Chart':

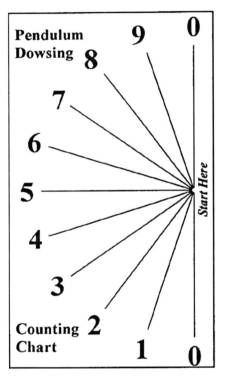

1. Hold your Pendulum over the 'Start Here'.
2. Ask your Pendulum to point to a number that you choose.
3. Check that your Pendulum makes a clockwise circle - to indicate 'OK'.
4. Check that it does point along the line of the number chosen.
5. Repeat with other numbers.

See where your Pendulum points when you choose a fractional number: like 3¼.

Pointing is a most useful way of using your Pendulum - so the amount of time that you spend on practice is not wasted.

Segment Selection

One of the benefits of pointing with your Pendulum is that you can make a segmented diagram, each segment identified with an option - such as writing the names of various places to go on holiday in each segment.

Then ask *"Which is the [best place for me to go on my next holiday] ?"* and see which is indicated by your Pendulum.

It is also best to label one segment as 'Other' - and if that segment is indicated, listen for the first thought that 'pops' into your Mind.

You can do this by holding it to one side and see where it points, or use your other hand to point with a pencil or your finger to items until your Pendulum gives a YES signal.

When you are given one selection, ask if there is also another to be found - you may have more than one error in a program, or need more than one supplement if you are checking what is needed for your good health.

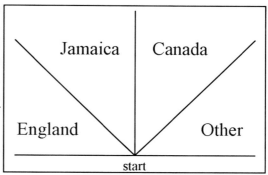

Your Handy Chart

Since most of us have two hands, we can use the spare one (the one not holding your Pendulum !) as a chart for many purposes.

It is best to use signals that conform to indicators that you see often, such as the speedometer and charging gauge of your car - your mind-brain team is accustomed to the signals used.

This is a quick way to check on your health or vitality, if medications are beneficial to you, how many tablets should be taken (dose, doses per day - these may change with effect already achieved), percentage accuracy of a statement, etc.

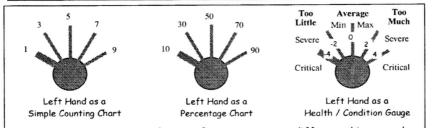

Left Hand as a
Simple Counting Chart

Left Hand as a
Percentage Chart

Left Hand as a
Health / Condition Gauge

You can use your ingenuity to let your fingers mean many different things - so long as you have ensured that your Mind-Brain team understands the meanings to be signalled for each 'hand-chart' - and that you have specified to your Mind-Brain team which 'hand-chart' is being used for the Dowsing you are now doing !

Locating and Evaluating Noxious Energies

Location of earth energies is best done by Dowsing - which works in all planes of existence, in all dimensions.

Accordingly I have designed a Logarithmic Numerical Chart specially for the Dowsing of the values encountered in handling noxious energies.

Unity (the value of 1.0 on the chart) represents the **'Average input of Beneficial Life Force/Energy that you receive in an hour from all sources'** - or 'Hourly Input' for short.

Extremely durable Vinyl-Plastic business cards printed with this chart are available (with a glass bead Pendulum) from the Holistic Intuition Society - to purchase one, see our web site: www.in2it.ca/tools.htm - or see our other contact information in this book.

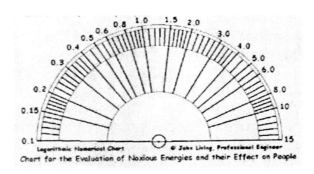

Logarithmic Numerical Chart © John Living, Professional Engineer
Chart for the Evaluation of Noxious Energies and their Effect on People

To use the chart, ask your Heart-Mind-Brain team to signal the amount of your 'Hourly Input' that would be used by you if you were to remain in the spot below the centre point of the card.

In most places this will be in the range from 0.2 to 0.4, signifying that it is a good position for you. Any value below 1.0 indicates that you have a net gain of beneficial energy, but the closer to 1.0 the less spare energy is available for other normal activities.

Any value greater than 1.0 means that you would have a net loss of energy if remaining in that place. The greater the value, the more detrimental is the noxious energy.

Any position giving a reading above 0.4 is best avoided.

You can go around your bed or chair (and elsewhere in the room) to get an idea of where the energy lines are running, and then plot the values on a sketch of the room to give you a 'map' of the energetic situation.

Using this map you can decide the best location for your chair or bed.

If you wish to identify the underlying causes of any noxious energy, you can ask your Heart to indicate YES or NO to the various types of causes.

The order of asking about depletion energies may best be:

1. Earthbound Energies (Souls, Spirits - of all types) - since they are so strong that their effect 'blankets out' other readings.
2. Curses - because they are usually covering a very large area.
3. EMF Radiations - often being noxious over a large area (from transformers), or very local (electric appliances).
4. Noxious Water Veins - they wander across the grids.
5. Curry Lines - easily identifiable, known spacing.
6. Pollution in Hartmann Grid - perhaps more common in rural areas, due to unbalanced electrical distribution systems.
7. Other Sources - and ask as guided by your Intuition.

Remember that there may be more than one type of energy that is noxious for you.

Methods of Transmuting Noxious Energies

There are very simple, exceedingly effective, and remarkably inexpensive ways to transmute noxious energies to become beneficial.

Earthbound Energies

If you get a reading of 5 or more at any point, it may be the effect of a 'Lost Soul' - so ask your Heart to get Angelic Assistance for the Lost Soul - to escort them to Heaven, or take any other appropriate action.

Then ask your Heart if this has been done, and if so then recheck the values at that place - they may well now be at normal good levels.

Curses

These may not have been placed intentionally ! Just 'wishing' that 'something bad' happen to a person, family, or community could be the cause. This may have happened many centuries (or even millennia) ago, and the person who placed the curse may have departed.

The energies involved in any curse do not like their job, but are 'stuck with it' since nobody has freed them. This is a job that you can do very easily - just tell *"All involved in all curses of all __times__ on this land and buildings are now free ! So now go 'into the Light' !"* and ask the Angelic Forces to help them on their way. Note 'times' is plural !

EMF Radiations

Gary Skillen, a past president of the Canadian Society of Dowsers, has found that crushed calcite crystals are excellent for absorbing the EMF radiations.

I experimented with placing thought forms of such crystals at a few electrical outlets and in front of my sound system, and found that they worked well; but after a couple of days the effect returned, so I asked why this happened. I was told *"We are overloaded. We need to be grounded."* - so I placed a grounding thought form in the piles of metaphysical calcite crystals, and they are doing a good job again.

The effectiveness of the calcite crystals seems to be enhanced by placing a sodalite crystal on top; if you placed a thought form of calcite crystals, then use another thought form for the sodalite (or add it to the calcite thought form).

How do you place a 'Thought Form' ? You just picture it being built - using your Heart-Mind-Brain team ! You explain the job, the length of time for the job to be done, charge the energies involved to do the job by sending them 'True Holy Love', and send your gratitude and thanks to all involved in this task.

Ray Machell reports on his testing of this method:

"The first item to be cleared was my new 21" computer monitor. Before starting I measured the distance that the monitor radiated energy that was detrimental to me. It was 64", much more than I expected.

With thought I placed crushed calcite crystals around the base, the edges of the screen, and on top of the monitor.

Measurement showed that the radiation had been reduced to 40".

I then imagined a sodalite crystal on top of each pile of calcite crystals - the radiation was now reduced to only 18" !

I then grounded each pile of crystals by thinking that each was connected by wire to an imaginary ground rod driven into the earth. Incredible - the radiation was now only $2\frac{1}{2}$" !!

In all this procedure I asked permission by Dowsing to do the work, indicated the purpose of the request and the length of time needed to be effective - in this case the time that I owned the monitor.

Upon completion, I gave thanks to all involved."

Noxious Water Veins

These seem to be noxious because they get loaded with 'bad thoughts' - water is very receptive to thoughts, as demonstrated by Dr Emoto in his book 'Message from Water', which shows the various patterns formed in ice crystals when subjected to written notes, different types of music, and homeopathic remedies.

First locate the vein of water running deep below your room, and find the direction of flow - also by Dowsing - just ask !

Now go as far upstream as possible, and bless the vein and the water that it carries:"*I Bless with 'True Holy Love' this water vein and all the water that it carries, and ask the help of 'The System' and the 'Angelic Forces' to Heal this water vein and all the water that it carries for all time, and to change its effect to become beneficial for all life.*"

Curry Lines

These may not be seen by clairvoyants, so are often ignored by people who rely on their 'second sight', which seems to operate in the 'Astral Plane'.

The Curry Grid exists in a higher plane of existence - but has effect on lower planes.

The grid runs NW-SE and NE-SW, the grid lines alternating YIN and YANG, forming vortices (like miniature tornados) at the grid junctions.

The strength of the lines varies, similar to a city's road system - most being like residential roads with acceptable strength, with collector roads at intervals which can be noxious, and with occasional highways of very high noxicity. If you sleep on a highway, expect to get 'run over' !

To Heal these Curry lines, Bless them in a similar way to the Blessing for noxious water veins.

As an example, the following was reported by Gary Skillen:

While teaching how to locate these zones we identified a Curry crossing point.

Each student took turns to stand on the point and described the effect on their bodies. Some felt sick to their stomachs, others tipped over or got a tingling sensation.

Suddenly a thought came to me to use my Dowsing to find out how detrimental this crossing was to humans.

On a scale from 1 (no problem) to 10 (most detrimental) this crossing was at 10. My next thought was:

"Maybe this Curry line has its own consciousness, its own awareness of itself; and is suffering as well ! And if I acknowledge the fact that it has its own awareness with respect, perhaps I can communicate with the energies involved".

I then asked:

"Are you detrimental to your own self ?" YES

"Do you want to remain detrimental ?" NO

"Do you want to change to being beneficial ?" YES

"Do I have permission to help you change to being beneficial ?" YES

"So be it !"

I took my Pendulum and allowed it to swing in the direction necessary to make the change - it swung clockwise for about 2 to 3 minutes, and then stopped.

I asked *"Is the correction made ?"* YES.

Each student then took turns standing on the same spot and reporting how they felt - some were apprehensive about repeating their previous experience, but all were pleasantly surprised !

This same crossing point now gave them more energy - and it was beneficial !

Pollution in Hartmann Grid
This seems to be caused by 'out of balance' electrical currents that are using the ground as their return path to 'source', and are most noticeable in rural areas.

I suggest that you treat them in the same way as other EMF energies, using grounded thought forms of calcite and sodalite. Metal rods driven into their flow path may also be used to divert the flow - or even the placing of thought forms instead of real ones !

An alternative way is to place a thought form of a solid 'Good Gold' ring around the house, to act as a 'traffic circle' for the enegies involved. This method may also be used for energies in the Curry Grid - using a separate ring.

If using these methods, the intent that you have must be clearly expressed, in a similar fashion to the Blessing of noxious water veins.

Pendulum Power
One aspect of using a Pendulum that is not often realized is its ability to magnify thoughts. When a Pendulum makes a circle (as in your YES and NO signals) the form created by your hand, string and the Pendulum is a cone - a circular pyramid.

Pyramids have long been recognized as having a special effect on energies due to their shape - even sharpening razor blades, and mummifying any meat product that they contain.

This effect is used in the normal loud speakers attached to your sound system - a magnet is vibrated by your amplifier, and its vibrations are magnified by the paper cone to which it is attached.

Your Pendulum acts in exactly the same way to magnify your thoughts !

So when you use your Pendulum to Bless a Curry line or noxious water vein the effect is just much stronger and more effective.

When using your Pendulum always be sincere - as in Prayer; you are working with the 'God Energy' and 'Angelic Forces'.

Blessing Food

It is probably true that the value to you of the food that you eat can be measured by its aura - the 'Life Radiance' that it has. So if you can increase such radiance, the food will be more beneficial for you.

Experiment

1. Measure the aura of your food (feel or Dowse for it).
2. Bless your food and measure again - it will have expanded.
3. Bless again using your Pendulum - any further increase ?

Repeat on more food (or next time you eat) this time Blessing with 'Blessing 995' - it may be even more effective !

More Dowsing

There is much more to using your Intuition - and improving your Intuitive skills by Dowsing. If you are interested in so being able to improve life for yourself, your family, and your friends then see the book 'Intuition Technology' - available from the Holistic Intuition Society.

In today's world, the skill of Dowsing is used more in Healing and maintaining wellness than in the traditional search for water. This includes selecting vitamins and supplements - and the most suitable brands and the dosages needed.

Kinesiology, where a Healer tests a patient, is used for many forms of diagnosis - including the identification of items to which the patient is allergic.

Dowsing can also be used for locating lost (or stolen) items, mineral deposits, and missing people or pets. Make certain that harm is not caused to any life form in all work that you do, and remember that one of the laws of life is that what you send to others comes back to you, multiplied, and perhaps in different ways.

A list of Dowsing societies in English speaking countries is included - you can contact these societies for help from experienced Dowsers who are in your area, and you may find that they have a chapter within easy travel distance.

Meeting with other Dowsers is always fun, and you can learn from each other. If you cannot meet in person, then you may find the Dowsing email groups a good way to share views and experiences.

Physicians

Most people who go to a medical school do so because they want to help others to be healthy - very few just because of the money involved.

The teaching at medical schools is focused on the recognition of symptoms, identification of illness, and treatment - usually by prescription of drugs considered to be appropriate.

In daily practice the physician is often faced with situations which are not clear and precise - one or more problems may exist, and usually the physician uses Intuition to decide how to proceed.

I am sure that most physicians will completely agree that this is the case - and that the more successful physicians are those who rely on their Intuitive abilities to augment their logical assessments.

Some physicians may just have an 'Intuitive Knowing' - others may need a method of accessing their Intuition 'On Demand' for the benefit of their patients, often a variation of 'Deviceless Dowsing'.

The first President of the Holistic Intuition Society was a retired medical doctor of high repute, who had been a member of the Dowsing Societies in America, Britain, and Canada.

He told me that he used his Pendulum (under the desk, where it was hidden from view) to guide his diagnoses and selection of treatment, with great success in helping his patients.

The late Don Brannigan, MD, many times Mayor of Whitehorse, used his Pendulum in full view - and was hauled before the Yukon Medical Council on a number of occasions; he won his case each time, but the financial cost of legal assistance was enormous.

It seems that all this occurs because Dowsing is associated with 'weird forces' (such as 'water witching') instead of being recognized as a means of accessing Intuition - which is a natural gift given to all people, and can be developed and used for the benefit of all.

All physicians would give better care to their patients if they are aware of the existence and effect of noxious energies, if they would use their Intuition to see if these are troubling a particular patient, and if so would advise the patient to get help to check out the areas where s/he sleeps or sits for a long time.

As explained in this book, this may enable their treatments to be more effective - for the benefit of their patients.

Other Healers

Many people in the Healing Professions such as Naturopaths, Nurses, Acupuncturists, and Chiropractors work with the energy fields in and around a human body - and many use their awareness of the differences in these fields, assisted by their Intuition, to give their patients appropriate treatment.

It is becoming more accepted that problems appear in the auras of people before an illness shows itself in the physical body. This is an area that is generally ignored by the western medical systems - and results in enormous costs of treatment to deal with the illness.

Much of this expense may be eliminated if more credence was given to the use of Intuition by Healers (including Clairvoyants and Dowsers) who can locate, identify, and heal these problems in the very early stages.

Pharmaceutical Corporations

About 75% of all the Pharmaceutical drugs are plant based; the effective chemicals are identified and then extracted, often using toxic compounds in this process, which increase the danger from side effects.

Many are reconstituted from chemicals to match those found in plants; there is one big difference, however - the medicine from plants themselves have a life force, missing from manufactured medicines.

Recognizing the growing demand for natural medicines, the drug companies are making big efforts to buy-out the producers of natural medicines, and also lobbying hard (and with unfortunate success) to ban all natural medicines that are not produced by them - including vitamins and other supplements.

These companies have a proven history of manipulating research results used to obtain approvals, and it should not come as a surprise that many senior persons in the approval organizations eventually leave these positions for ones with the drug companies that pay far more. Does this indicate corruption in high places ?

In the United States of America the 'Morbidity and Mortality Report' of 9th. February, 2007 from the Centers for Disease Control and Prevention states that deaths from prescription drugs almost doubled between 1999 and 2004.

Comments made on this report include:

"Today's pharmaceutical industry is a massive fraud being perpetuated against the American people, propped up by illegal trade practices, monopolistic behaviour, and outright criminal behaviour on the part of the FDA". (See Nexus Magazine 14/3)

From a 'BizNez' perspective, a person who is cured is a lost sales opportunity - and side effects increase the market for drugs.

Dr Scott-Mumby, who wrote the foreword, comments (May 2007):

"Do children's psychology issues concern anybody ? They should. Some kids are on 2 and 3 heavy anti-depressive drugs. Real medical science ? Or killing kids for the sake of a few stinking dollars ?"

Health Organization

It seems that the pharmaceutical industry has managed to get a 'vast grip' on the various medical associations, which in turn have great influence on the Ministries of Governments in most countries.

A more holistic approach would improve Health and reduce the current massive expenditures - expected to grow in the future.

This needs our elected representatives to really understand the effects of the stranglehold now exerted by the Pharmaceutical Industry and the Medical Associations, and to be determined to make major changes in the Health Care Systems that now exist - for the benefit of all people, and at a reduced cost.

More recognition is needed of the non-physical systems of the Human Being, and of the skills available from energy workers to work with these systems of energy - including Intuition in general, and Dowsing in particular.

Perhaps if all Healing was included in Health Care benefits, and full records were kept of the resulting effectiveness, then the valuable contributions that energy workers can provide would be better appreciated - and Health Care improved.

In Closing - Many other problems, not just cancer, are attributable to some large degree to earth energies that are noxious to humans.

By eliminating the effects of these we can expect improvements in education and in behaviour, reductions in work losses and medical expenses, and better health at minimal cost.

Namaste   *John Living*

English Speaking Dowsing Organizations

Note to this edition

The previous editions made lists of books, reference, source material, and societies which were mainly German. The English translations of these titles have been included in the main text, but are omitted from this list. If needed, reference should be made to the original German editions of Käthe Bachler's work.

See www.in2it.ca for current addresses and internet connections.

Australia
Dowsers Society of New South Wales
7 Maycock St, Denistone East, NSW
        www.divstrat.com.au   dsnsw@yahoo.com.au

Dowsing Society of Victoria
PO Box 4278, Ringwood, VIC 3134
        www.dsv.org.au

Dowsers' Club of South Australia Inc
PO Box 2427, Kent Town 5071, South Australia.

North Tasmania Dowsing Association
2515 West Tamar Highway, Exeter, Tasmania 7275, Australia.

South Tasmania Dowsing Association
PO Box 530, Moonah, Tasmania 7009, Australia

Canada
Canadian Society of Dowsers (Ontario and eastern Canada)
Suite 152, #7 - 800 Queenstown Rd, Stoney Creek, ON L8G 1A7
        www.canadiandowsers.org   1-888-588-8958

Canadian Society of Questers (Prairies and British Columbia)
PO Box 4873, Vancouver, BC V6B 4A6
        www.questers.ca   (604) 944-8683

India
Indian Society of Dowsers   Arun Patel (President)
81/961 Shreenath apartment, Nr Vayash Wadi,
        Nava Vadaj, Ahemadabad 380 013, Gujarat, India

Ireland
Society of Irish Dowsers
31 Ardmore Grove, Artane, Dublin 5
    www.irishdiviners.com

New Zealand
New Zealand Society of Dowsing and Radionics
PO Box 41-095, St Luke's SQ, Mt. Albert, Auckland 1030
    www.dowsingnewzealand.org

United Kingdom
British Society of Dowsers

2 St. Ann's Road, Malvern, Worcestershire, WR14 4RG
    www.britishdowsers.org   44 01624 576969
    info@britishdowsers.org

United States of America
American Society of Dowsers

P.O. Box 24, Danville, VT 05828-0024, USA
    www.dowsers.org   (802) 684-3417
    asd@dowsers.org

Ozark Research Institute
PO Box 387, Fayetteville, AR 72702-0387
    www.ozarkresearch.org   (479) 582-9197

Email Lists open to all who are interested in Dowsing

International Society of Dowsers
Purely web based - www.internationaldowsers.org
To join, go to: www.groups.yahoo.com/group/digital-dowsers/join
(Note: a Yahoo! ID is required)
Or email: digital-dowsers-subscribe@yahoogroups.com - no message needed.

ASD Digital Dowsers
is an online cyber chapter of ASD meeting round the clock, planet wide.
To join, see: www.photon.cc/mailman/listinfo/digitaldowsers
Membership of American Society of Dowsers is NOT required !

Other books by John Living

Intuition 'On Demand'

We look at the way that our beings operate, including an overview of our 'energy bodies' and 'soul senses', and how to work with our Heart as our link to 'Upstairs'.

We examine the methods used to liaise with our sub-conscious self to improve our working relationship, and how awareness of our environment and expansion of our knowledge increase our abilities to work with our Intuition.

We are 'ruled' by our beliefs; some are based on things that we have been told by others - that may not be 'our truth'. But these become established as programs that we run automatically.

Examples are given of ways to change now existing programs, and how to install new programs for our well-being.

Some very simple ways to improve our health are discussed, and methods of helping our Heart-Mind-Brain team to access our Intuition and to signal answers via our nervous-muscular system are examined, including the use of our real physical '6th sense' - the sense of balance.

We investigate methods of amplifying our Intuitive signals to enable more diverse use of our 'Power of Thought', including effective ways of improving life for all by adjusting the vibrational patterns of energy - including the use of thought to make simple medicine for oneself !

At the end of the book some interesting games are described which will help participants to improve their Intuitive abilities.

The approach used in this book is to 'keep it simple'. There are a lot of little hints - if they suit you, then use them to improve your life.

These 'snippets' are not repeated endlessly, so you will probably have to read the book a few times to get the best value from them.

Intuition Technology

This book was originally written as a text book for a weekend course; the appendices included important information that could not be covered in just one weekend !

Hundreds of copies have been sold, with much positive feed-back - and not one complaint !

The book has now been re-written so that the content is not constrained by a time factor - the material can be studied at leisure.

The essential 'stuff' of this book is that we all have Intuition, and our Heart-Mind-Brain team provides the best linkage to our Intuition - giving signals via our nervous-muscular system.

This method of accessing our Intuition 'On Demand' is also called 'Dowsing' - a term which is perceived by some as having negative connotations. We explain why this is so, and why it is not true.

The skills taught in this book have been used for a great many years - mainly to help others. There are many wonderful teachers around the globe, and this book tries to collect their wisdom together.

The book starts from scratch - teaching basic skills, and then showing how these can be used for the good of all. Even experienced Dowsers have gained from reading this book - since some aspects have not previously been explained in simple terms.

In the past Dowsing has been used mainly to locate water wells, and sometimes minerals. The major use today is in health matters - locating noxious energies and Healing them; identifying health problems and finding ways to overcome them; and improving the well-ness of people by using our 'Power of Thought'.

Another aspect of Dowsing is its use for accessing information; ways to get help from the 'Universal Knowledge Banks' are described, so that we can make better decisions - or, like Albert Einstein (a Dowser who so obtained his theory of relativity) be able to develop new ways of 'doing things' due to our improved understanding.

As a basis, we try to describe how 'All things Are' - including the work done by C.W.Leadbeater and Annie Besant between 1895 and

1932 in describing sub-sub-sub atomic particles. They were, of course, ridiculed - since there could not be anything smaller than an atom !

Everything that exists is made of energy - and this applies to other dimensions as well as the physical dimensions. Knowing this, we can understand how to work with 'All That Is' for the general good.

Understanding the 'Power of Thought' and how 'We are all the same' gives us the ability to work with these energies and to Heal them as needed.

This includes the use of Radionics machines - how to make and use simple ones drawn of paper that work even better than the mechanical machines that cost so much.

Map Dowsing is taught - including the mapping of water veins at distant locations and the mapping of energies around a life form such as humans, animals, and plants.

More and more Healers are recognizing that problems are found in the auras of a life form before a disease manifests in the physical body.

Western medicine seeks mainly to stop the effects of a disease - rarely to uncover and Heal the underlying causes, which are often not in the physical dimension.

This book delves into the many complicated systems that exist within and work with the human body, and suggests Healing methods that can be very effective.

Energy Healing, using Dowsing, can locate and identify these causes, and Heal them before disease manifests in the physical body.

Many Healers seem to be attacked - the reasons for this is discussed, and methods suggested to protect oneself and Heal the energies causing the attacks so that they become beneficial !

The techniques taught in this book cannot hurt anyone - but can help people to create a better and more healthy life, for themselves and for others !

Miracles do happen when we work with 'Upstairs' having the intent of helping others with 'True Holy Love'.

The Holistic Intuition Society's 'Shop'

"Love Living" Bracelets

Background

In the 1925 Georges Lakhovsky in France developed a coil for the protection of trees; copper wire was stuck into the ground, turns were made around the tree, and the loose end was pointed towards the sky as an aerial. In 1928 he formed a variation of this that was geared to improve the health of humans, which he called the 'multi-wave oscillator', based on his then new theory that cells are microscopic oscillating circuits.

This was successfully used in French, Italian, and Swedish clinics, and when Lakhovsky escaped to the USA in 1941 it proved successful in a major New York hospital. Among problems successfully treated were cancerous growths from Radium burns, goiters, arthritis, chronic bronchitis, congenital hip dislocation, and many others. (Tompkins & Bird: 'Secret Life of Plants').

Design of the Rings

John Living made a number of different rings, testing the effect on glasses of water showed that the water had a radiance of about 5KÅ (5,000 Ångstroms - the human body for a normal person is about 6.5 KÅ) which in 2 minutes increased to 20KÅ for the medium sized rings and 60 KÅ for the smallest ring - the effect is more concentrated.

They are sturdy, attractive, and within the reach of most purses. So which ring type is best ? This depends on the use !

The bracelets and smaller rings #1, #2, and #3 are of twisted copper wire, having a small gap; a vinyl tube prevents the copper from being in direct contact with your skin.

They give your blood the vibrational pattern of copper, similar to the way a homeopathic remedy works.

This waterproof casing design permits easy cleaning, prevents corrosion, and allows opening. These rings can be worn, or used to energize foods and drinks. The medium ring, #6, is similar - it fits on most chairs for you to sit on.

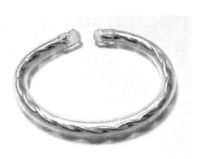

The larger rings, #8, #10, and #12, are of 1/4 inch diameter copper tube (for increased sturdiness) having a twisted wire connector in the gap to encourage clockwise rotation of the energies in the tube.

They are intended for healing the energies in a body and in its aura.

The vinyl encased copper bracelet is sealed watertight, for easy washing, and the combination of vinyl with copper blends into the skin colour, so that the bracelet is less noticeable. A hardy bracelet, suitable for constant wear, even ideal for a man in the office or working outside.

Using the Rings

The strongest effect is in the plane of the ring. It seems that 'not good' energies cannot exist inside the ring; the effect is also 'transmitted' in a column above and below this plane, expanding at 45° and reducing in intensity as the distance increases.

To find which size LOVE LIVING bracelet fits you:

Measure around your ankle / wrist with a tape measure send it to us, and we will send you the correct size .

Wear your bracelet loosely - leave about 1/2 to 1 inch gap between the ends.

You can expect all the water in your body (over 75% of you !) to become potentized with a high radiance.

Germs and viruses do not thrive in such an environment, so your LOVE LIVING Bracelets helps to keep you healthy !

A number of successes are reported with the relief of headaches by placing a #2 Energy ring around the neck - if below a shirt or sweater, it is not noticeable.

It may be that some people who have other head problems, perhaps including Alzheimer's and Parkinson's diseases, benefit from wearing a neck ring. The cost of a trial is minimal, the possible benefits considerable, and there is no health risk involved.

A Simple Test you can do yourself

Put water from the same source into 2 glasses and put one glass into your 'LOVE LIVING' Energy Ring. After 10 minutes taste each glass. Repeat at 20 minutes and 30 minutes.

You can expect the untreated water to retain its original taste, while the taste of the treated water improves.

At the same time you can use an Aurameter (or other Dowsing tool) to check the location of the aura of the water; you will find that the aura of the treated water expands !

The Ptah Pendulum

John Living found that the Osiris Pendulum has a special ability to locate 'not good' energies in a person's aura, and when used in 'extraction mode' (an anti-clockwise circle) it removed such energies.

But there was a problem - they tended to go into the hand of the Healer/Dowser who was using the Pendulum !

To overcome this, John attached his Osiris Pendulum to the 'extract' end of one of the Healing Coils developed by Slim Spurling.

This converted the energies that were removed into being 'good' energies - and thus prevented deleterious effects from being experienced by the Healer/Dowser, giving instead a beneficial effect.

The next step was to attach one of Slim's Coils to a cord, so as to make a Pendulum. This was even more powerful in extracting 'not good' energies and converting them to being 'good', but did not have the ability of the Osiris Pendulum in locating problems in auras.

An effort was made to get the Osiris Pendulum, designed on geometric theory, to teach the 'Slim's Coil' Pendulum its skill in locating problems in auras - and this was successful !

The Isis Pendulum has the gift of putting 'good' energies into the recipient in a similar way, so a cord was attached to the output end of one of Slim's Coils to make a Pendulum that put 'good' energy into a person - and again this was a success !

Then the thought was received "Why not combine them into a dual purpose Pendulum ?" - and so the 'Ptah Pendulum' was developed.

John Living has tested this on himself and on a number of other people who needed Healing - with excellent results.

He has used it to locate and Heal 'not good' energies in the land, such as curses and other 'bad medicine', and understands that it is one of the most powerful Healing devices that exists.

When working with the Healing Angels and other Healing Energies John uses the 'Ptah Pendulum' to clear energies that are causing problems as a preliminary step to reduce the work needed to be done by the Healing Energies / Angels.

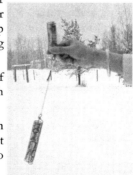

All the 'Ptah Pendulums' are blessed with the abilities of the Osiris and Isis Pendulums, and have been made with True Holy Love.

The picture shows an early version - we now produce an improved version made of tinned copper wire to prevent tarnishing, and with a chain having swivels at each end to eliminate twisting.

Signals

In all work with the 'Ptah Pendulum' a clockwise circle indicates YES and is the 'Input Mode'. An anti-clockwise circle indicates NO and is the 'Extract Mode'.

When asking a question it does not matter which end of the Pendulum is held.

The 'Ptah Pendulum' will extract or input, and then swing towards the next position that it needs to go - the direction could be one of two ways, since it is swinging, and your Intuition will guide you to the correct place.

If you go in the wrong direction, the 'Ptah Pendulum' will not circle (or make a very small signal) - so reverse the direction that you are moving the Pendulum. When in the correct place it will circle to do the needed work.

Holding your 'Ptah Pendulum'

In extract mode, the hand holds the shorter of the two coils. For input mode, the longer coil is held. To avoid bending the coil that is held, hold it at its bottom - the strain is not transmitted to the part of the coil above your hand.

Start at the head of the person or centre of the token, and make an anti-clockwise circle (extract mode, shorter coil in hand) around this point, widening in a spiral to enclose most of the Healee; then hold the 'Ptah Pendulum' stationary at the start point - it will start to circle on its own accord to extract 'not good' energies.

When the circling finishes, the 'Ptah Pendulum' will swing, pointing to the next location of 'not good' energies - move it slowly in the direction indicated until it starts to swing again. This is repeated until it remains stationary.

Now change to input mode - the longer coil is held in hand, making clockwise circles - again on its own accord - and this procedure is repeated.

Logically this should remove all 'not good' energies, and replace them all with 'good' energies. But the metaphysical world is not logical !

Perhaps what happens is that some 'not good' energies resist the extraction, but are weakened by the input of True Holy Love, so that by repeating this whole procedure again more 'not good' energies will be extracted.

To make certain that all has been cleared, keep on repeating the extraction mode and then input mode until no circling occurs. And as a final check, start again at the start point and make a spiral, then go to the start point and sees if any swinging or circling occurs.

If so, then repeat the whole procedure again - and keep on until there is not any swinging or circling.

Note that this is not just to Heal people - for 'person' you can substitute 'animal', 'bird', etc.

'L' Rods

These are made from welding rods, with a wooden handle having a plastic insert for low friction movement and a metal end cap.

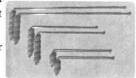

The rod arm has a metal end cap to enhance your Dowsing response and prevent damage to people.

Glass Bead Pendulums

The glass beads have been hand made by craftsmen, and come in various colours and configurations; they are held by a braided nylon string, the string colour being suitable for the bead.

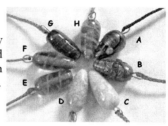

Bendable Bobber

This tool has pewter weights fitted to the end of a specially wound spring 'wand' inserted into a ball-point pen case. It gives great sensitivity, and bends to fit in your pocket.

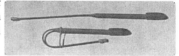

DVDs of Speakers and Workshops

We have recorded the lectures and workshops on Dowsing and on Healing at the conventions promoted by the Society, and have these available on DVDs that are playable world-wide.

The workshops were given by recognized masters of Dowsing to teach their skills - including the ability of Dowsers to use their 'Power of Thought' for healing the energies of humans, animals, and plants.

More Information

The Holistic Intuition Society sells more Dowsing and Healing tools - these are shown on our website at: **www.in2it.ca/tools.htm** together with prices and ordering information.

The key intent is to provide simple tools that can be easily used, at reasonable cost, and that do their job effectively and safely without any side effects.

The Holistic Intuition Society

c/o Executive Secretary: John Living, Professional .Engineer
RR# 1 S9 C6, Galiano Island, BC, V0N 1P0 Canada
Telephone (250)539-5807 Toll Free Canada & USA: 1-866-369-7464

**Unfortunately we cannot process credit cards - except by PayPal
PayPal is set-up on our web site,
A cheque or money order in Canadian or US funds is acceptable.**

Printed in the United States
148474LV00002B/4/P

9 780968 632352